THE REST OF YOUR LIFE IS THE BEST OF YOUR LIFE

*David Brown's Guide to
Growing Gray Disgracefully*

THE REST OF YOUR LIFE IS THE BEST OF YOUR LIFE

David Brown's Guide to Growing Gray Disgracefully

BARRICADE BOOKS INC.
FORT LEE, NEW JERSEY

Published by
Barricade Books Inc.
1530 Palisade Avenue
Fort Lee, N.J. 07024

Portions of this book appeared in *Brown's Guide to Growing Gray*,
published in 1987 by Delacorte Press

Library of Congress Cataloging-in-Publication Data:

Brown, David, 1916-
    The rest of your life is the best of your life : Brown's guide to
growing gray / David Brown.
        p.   cm.
    Rev. ed. of: Brown's guide to growing gray. c1987.
    ISBN 0-942637-35-6
    1. Aged men—Health and Hygiene. 2. Aging. 3. Rejuvenation.
I. Brown, David, 1916- Brown's guide to growing gray. II. Title.
RA777.8.B78   1991
646.7′9—dc20
                                                           91-19324
                                                                CIP

MANUFACTURED IN THE UNITED STATES OF AMERICA

For Helen, my raison d'être

CONTENTS

Contents

PREFATORY NOTE

This little book is not intended to be the definitive work on staying young. It will become apparent, one hopes not too painfully, that it is not rooted in extensive research, statistical analysis, and the like. It is instead a collage of wholly personal convictions on mastering the art of seeming never to grow old. While conceivably written from an elitest point of view, what I have set down is, I believe, applicable to almost anyone who is over fifty or hopes to be.

One other caveat. It is obviously written for men. However, much of it does, I think, also apply to women, especially the new and growing group of independent women. I hope they all profit from this book—because if they profit I will too.

—DAVID BROWN

FOREWORD

Don't Stop. Start!

One afternoon at a Dutch Treat Club lunch in New York, a publisher named Bernard Geis asked what I was doing with my life. It was a polite, bread-breaking question.

I told him that at 70 I was busier than at 35, producing four movies, a television series, three plays on Broadway and one in London.

Geis exclaimed, "My God, why don't you write a book!" I did. Apparently it changed some people's lives.

Readers ranging from Baron Guy de Rothschild to my local postman said it gave them a new perspective on living. Hollywood star Warren Beatty, although too young for its message, proclaimed the book his "bible." Auto tycoon Victor Potamkin bought hundreds of copies for friends as did super agent Irving "Swifty" Lazar, never busier than in his eighties. A media personality famed for his stalwart, powerhouse persona told me it was his prescription for the depression and symptoms of burn-out that too often afflicted him.

There's more. Wives gave copies to their husbands (although they might not have, had they read it). Mistresses (who *had* read it) placed it at their bedside (their lovers told me). And unstuffy daughters thought it would make a dandy Father's Day present (even knowing their mothers might disapprove).

Obviously, the book touched multiple nerves of young and old. It suggested that the last years of life can be the best, the sexiest, the wealthiest and the healthiest.

The years between 65 and 75 have been the best years of my life; best for work, best for making money, best for making love although less is more in that category.

Perhaps you think I didn't have much fun in my early years. Not so. I gorged myself on youthful pleasures. As the book reveals, I fell in love—often. I drank—too much. I smoked cigars, leaving clouds of fragrant Havana in my wake.

And yet, as Alan J. Lerner melodically put it, *I'm glad I'm not young anymore*. Youth is too fragile, easily intimidated, unsure of itself.

I no longer suffer the pain of needing to be liked. I like myself—popular where it counts. I say and do what I want without worrying much what others think.

Facing your own mortality in five, ten, fifteen years or minutes you no longer care what some pipsqueak says or writes about you. "Fugum," as Norman Mailer used to say.

I have written this updated, completely revised edition of my book to show new readers and old what has worked for me in my mid-seventies. It *can* work for you, although I make no representation that it will work for everyone. You have to want not to succumb to being out of it, terminally bored, wondering where life went. Life went thataway and you can still find it if you really try. I'm saddened to meet men of my age or even younger who have given up, whose mental and physical responses are faltering, who have no vigor or virility. You can get it all back but you must go for it now.

My book will tell you how I got through the thickets of sex, money, work, marriage, divorce, memory lapses, friendships, depression and fear of death. It contains nearly everything I've learned in more than seventy years. When I was a young man, the number one best seller was *Life Begins at Forty* by Walter B. Pitkin. *Forty*? Today puberty begins at forty. Life begins at sixty, seventy or eighty if you work at it. Whatever *your* age, don't stop. Start!

CHAPTER ONE

Work Yourself to Death— It's the Only Way to Live

My friend, fabled literary agent Irving "Swifty" Lazar, is eighty-two years old. He recently told me that he woke up one morning, thinking, "If I didn't have something to do today, I'd rather be dead."

If you don't have something to do today, you *are* dead. You are not only dead but are also in a purgatory of boredom. Nobody needs you. No matter how your bones creak or what difficulty you have getting out of bed, I recommend that you work yourself to death. It's the only way to live.

Years ago, I had the good luck to have made enough money never to have to work again. I was tempted by the idea. I tried spending seven days without responsibility, duties, or deadlines at an island resort in the Caribbean. Within hours I was consulting airline schedules back to snowy Manhattan. Today when somebody, seeing me at five in the morning on a remote film location, asks why I still work, my standard reply is "If I didn't, who would have lunch with me?"

Easy Street is a dead end. So are stressless jobs. Some time back, my wife and I stopped over in Fiji en route to Australia (to work). I asked our Fijian driver what it was like to live in a tropical paradise where there is always enough food, never a cold day, and even the sharks don't bother to bite (they're so overfed). "Mister," declared the driver, "my dream is to drive a taxi in Chicago."

Almost everybody I know who feels young, vital, and sexy—no matter what his age—is working. If he's been retired because of company policy, he has gone off to other, and often more arduous, work. In his late-seventies, Victor Potamkin, the nation's largest Cadillac dealer, said, "I find that work is a great therapy. I think anybody who retires is crazy; when you retire, you're waiting to die." When Armand Hammer was in his late eighties he was making plans for his late nineties. Never mind that he didn't quite make it. Thinking he would kept him going. Robert Penn Warren became our first poet laureate at eighty. Martha Graham danced until she was 75 and choreographed until her death (from pneumonia) at 95. At this writing, one hundred-year-old Broadway director George Abbott, himself a bridegroom of only a decade or so, is planning a new production. George Burns says he is committed to play London's Palladium when he's a hundred. "How can I die when I'm booked?" he quips. The point is you won't die if you're "booked." So stay "booked."

My friend and former partner, Richard Zanuck, his wife, Lili, and I produced a movie titled *Cocoon*. The story takes place in a retirement home. We discovered that older actors we selected to play retirees—the likes of Hume Cronyn, Jessica Tandy, Jack Gilford, Maureen Stapleton, Don Ameche, Gwen Verdon—looked too young to play their own ages. They had to be aged with makeup, taught to limp and bend over. They had never stopped working and therefore had no time to grow old.

Neither had Tom Carvel, owner of an ice-cream empire and active almost to the time of his death in his eighties. His reply to a newspaper interviewer was as stormy as a rock star's. "'Retirement!' he screams. 'Why should I retire? I'm not working. You call this work? When you can get up seven days a week and do what you want to do and enjoy doing, that's not work. What's so pleasurable about watching TV shows and movies all day that show nothing but violence and car crashes? That's not the stuff that built this country.'"

The American dream of early retirement has turned out to be a nightmare. Consider this statement by Walter Kiechel III in a recent issue of *Fortune:* "Retirement, the experts say, seems to bring an increase in the incidence of suicide, alcoholism, and divorce." Dr. Jonas Salk, discoverer of the Salk polio vaccine, declares, ". . . looking forward to retirement and seeking to do nothing can be fatal." That's why, at seventy-eight, he's still active. Even the Soviet Institute of Gerontology reports, "Man could live longer if he were allowed to work longer." Meanwhile, advertisements of financial institutions urge men and women in their thirties—one even used a picture of a baby—to "plan now" for their retirement years. Dreadful idea. I agree one should "plan now," but for more *work* and less play.

Some men and women who have retired with lavish benefits are going back to work and others who are being forced into early retirement (often with financial indurements) are fighting it or going into business for themselves. Here are some conclusions from the *Fortune* article previously quoted: "An increasingly common alternative is retiring from the old job and then, after a sobering glimpse of the void, taking on a new one. A recent survey of retired presidents and chief executives of the largest U.S. companies, conducted by Russell Reynolds Associates, an executive search firm, found that sixty-one percent of the respondents had returned to work, the majority within six months of stepping down from the catbird seat.", Some even manage to stay in the catbird seat. More than eighty chief executive officers of Forbes 500 companies are over sixty-five.

When men and women *don't* go back to work, the results can be devastating. According to a government study the highest incidence of heart attacks among men occurs one year after they stop working. Even more startling, a Pan Am pilot, about to be retired in his middle fifties, told me that two years after retirement airline pilots had, for their ages, a mortality rate higher than the population as a whole. This is especially significant. Airline pilots are certifiably healthy to the day of their retirement because of physical examinations required every six months by the Federal Aviation Authority. Why, then, do many of them die after giving up their work? Can it be that the stress and sense of responsibility they experienced as pilots were essential to keeping them alive? I believe so. It's persuasive evidence that giving up work can be hazardous to your health.

I've seen their faces, the retired ones. I've watched these once vigorous and commanding men shuffling around the decks of round-the-world cruise ships. They have no interests, no passions. Their energy is gone. They are old because they have been brainwashed to act old, to play the part. In addition to the floating retirement homes, you also see the vacant faces of the retired ones in Palm Springs and Palm Beach, in St. Petersburg, in Sun City—wherever we have segregated them to "God's waiting rooms."

How much better if they had worked themselves to death, died on the job, been committed to something other than themselves until the last living moment. You can't blame them for accepting retirement. They were victims of society's cruelest con job, that being able not to work is a desirable state, the cheerful culmination of a lifetime's labor. They and we have been persuaded that retirement is part of the normal process of our lives.

It is not a new idea. Retirement at sixty-five was first invoked at the time of Bismarck, a hundred years ago, when few lived that long, and if they did, were in their dotage. A half century later, work life was still thought to end at sixty-five, the age Social Security payments would begin. The idea persists to this day despite changes in the mandatory retirement age and quantrum leaps in life expectancy. In fact, companies now offer "earlier retirement" packages to people in their fifties, and some public servants can retire at forty.

"If you didn't know how old you were, how old would you be?" That was the question attributed (among others) to the legendary black musician Eubie Blake, himself over a hundred and still working at the time of his death. One answer is that you would be as old as you behave. If you are still performing a vital function other than breathing, you will be younger than you actually are. "Swifty" Lazar says, "If something wonderful doesn't happen to me by noon [when he customarily wakes up—which is by itself wonderful], I make it happen."

Am I painting too pretty a picture of the possibilities of feeling young in later life? Whatever became of senility, deafness, failing eyesight, and other afflictions of advancing years? They're there, of course. Some of us will fall to disease (even as younger people do), although statistics reveal more than two thirds of Americans *over seventy-five* are in good health. Far more of us older ones—more than ever before—can enjoy years of physical health—but, I believe, only if we *do something* with our later lives. My father lived to eighty-seven but was made to retire at sixty-five. He wasted twenty years doing nothing, didn't have a failing day until boredom and a touch of pneumonia killed him. I believe he could have lived to a hundred if he had worked longer.

9

According to Dr. James F. Fries, associate professor of medicine at Stanford University, ". . . It is possible and reasonable to expect that one can maintain health and vitality at as close to full levels for as long as possible; then, the biology of the organism will take over . . . and, after a reasonably short period of time, senescence and death will follow. *In realistic terms, one expects this will take place at an average age of approximately 85, as compared with the present 74.6 life expectancy.*" That's for those now being born, but if you have already reached your sixties and seventies your life expectancy is well past eighty too. If you're younger, plan now for an active old age. Social Security and pension plans will never be able to support the hordes of "baby boomers" when they start turning sixty—with decades of life ahead of them.

You won't be alone if you continue on the job. Gil Millstein, former news editor of *NBC Nightly News*, worked until his seventies in what is considered a high-pressure, young man's field. Mike Wallace of *Sixty Minutes* and its executive producer, Don Hewitt, both signed new contracts that will take them into their mid-seventies. Betty Furness at seventy-four was consumer affairs spokesperson for NBC's *Today* show and Freddy de Cordova produced *The Tonight Show* until he was past eighty and the show quit on him. Bob Hope will never quit.

Isaac Asimov, one of America's most successful authors, at seventy is publishing a new book every three weeks. At sixty-five, he threw a nonretirement party for himself. He said in a recent essay, "If the world should suddenly end, I hope it would find me at work. To me, stopping is like being defeated . . . to quit [work] is to kill the spirit that gives life its meaning and worth." George Bernard Shaw, who did his best work in his later years, pronounced retirement as "a working definition of hell." A renowned Manhattan lawyer, Simon Rifkind, at ninety kept a full working schedule, including frequent trips all over the world.

As you may have surmised, I consider the Great Divide not between life and death but between working and not working. Anybody who has been unemployed will tell you that. I remember my own not infrequent spells of joblessness—watching from my apartment window the going-to-work crowds, feeling isolated from the real world as people piled into the subways and buses with someplace to go, where they were expected and needed.

My advice is to start planning your second career while you're still on your first one. Not everyone can go from one executive post to another, ignore corporate retirement edicts or layoffs due to economic slow-downs. You may have to step down financially and in perceived status. Planning to open a business—if you are providing a need—can be more satisfying than having a swimming pool full of perks. You're the boss. Nobody can fire you. It may be better than the job or profession from which you retired or were fired. Not everyone even likes the work he's done most of his life. In fact, there may be *more* people who have hated their jobs and looked *forward* to leaving it. If you are one, now is your opportunity to plan for something more agreeable and experience the *joy* of work.

When Richard Zanuck and I founded our own movie-production company after being thrown out of executive posts we thought we had for life, we decided that never again would we let our lives be controlled by others, although we had no assurance we could succeed on our own. If we had held on to our old jobs, I, as an over-sixty-five employee, would have had to retire by now, and I would be a reader and not a writer of this book.

I can't begin to suggest what business or job you can fill except to advise you to try to find something that *interests* you—be it work at a country inn, or starting up a newsstand, a messenger service, a fax center, a travel agency, a shopping guide, or whatever. In a book titled *Success Over Sixty*, Albert Myers and Christopher Anderson make excellent suggestions for second careers and list companies that favor older employees. Chances are best that you will excel at what you like to do most. Your first new job is to conduct your own market research to discover what's out there. Eventually you'll find what you like. The important thing is to get going now and not to stop trying.

CHAPTER TWO

Let a Woman in Your Life—
Preferably More than One

I've observed that those who stay young all their lives *never* stop being interested in women. Do you remember the old movie *Citizen Kane*? If so, you may recall the scene in which Kane's former general manager said that years ago he had watched a girl for scarcely a minute on a ferry boat and not a month had gone by that he hadn't thought of that girl.

I identify with that character. There is hardly a day or an hour when I am not aware of the women around me. I peer at whatever comely creatures are walking about. I'm good at looking at women in automobiles, too, and I can get a fix on them before they speed away.

Like the character in *Citizen Kane*, I'll probably never see any of them again, but I can conjure up the woman-of-the-day, the woman-of-the-month, and sometimes the woman-of-a-lifetime. I can also dip into my memory bank and remember girls I desired more than fifty years ago. They were early women-of-a-lifetime and they stir me to this day.

I don't believe you're not still interested in women at your age, even if you're long since happily wed. You may have retired from sexual awareness, but you can always go back to work. As with swimming, you never forget the strokes. Whether you're married or single, women friends can be a joy and a rejuvenation. I'm talking about women *plural*—not just one woman. One is too few, too stuffy, too niggardly, and too dangerous. She may mistake your concentration for commitment. In choosing more than one you can be selective. The ratio of single women over forty to men is staggering—in your favor but hurry. Statistics indicate that in another generation or two there may be *fewer* women! What if you're still around?? Not to worry, unless you're Methuselah. The glut of available women is still so great that polygamy has been suggested in serious quarters to correct the imbalance. I'm not suggesting you take on the imbalance personally, but I do suggest you find female friends. You can attract the best of those engaged in the Great American Manhunt, but you must do everything to interest and charm them, not drop out to talk or play cards with male cronies.

You may not be ready for an affair, nor may the one you find be willing to be your lover. There's a wide and satisfying area of in-between choices—in between "looking" and going to bed. Some of my best "affairs" went no further than a touch of hands or an intensely personal conversation on a night flight to London. I'm not foreclosing going to bed (it can happen if a relationship becomes overheated), but you need to be wise, gutsy, and guiltless to bring off infidelity without emotional fallout. Also lucky.

I think healthy men and women, regardless of other commitments, evaluate each other as sexual partners when they meet. Circumstances decide how far the relationship is likely to go. It needn't go too far. I find women don't want to be bedded as much as desired and admired. Desiring and admiring them are sometimes enough—and safer, particularly in these times. I know that makes me feel good . . . and young.

If *you* need more and are willing to accept the risks, it might be wise to follow the advice of the Hollywood screenwriter Herman Mankiewicz, who counseled, "Never sleep with anyone who has more trouble or less money than you have."

To which I would add, never sleep with anyone whose sexual history is totally unknown to you (widows and recent divorcees are safest).

Even if she passes these tests and you are free to pursue the relationship, serious romance is hard work. You have to shape up and take pride in your appearance. You lose or gain weight, whichever is required. You dye your hair, cap your teeth, straighten your back, and, on occasion, your vital organ. You're jealous, wondering if there's someone else in her life. You experience feelings—some of them painful—you haven't had in years. But you're alive! Alive, that is, if you're not married; only a single man could get away with this transformation without arousing suspicion.

How about your ability to perform? Can you still get it up? Groucho Marx, confiding to a chum that he was about to have an affair, remarked, "I guess I'll bend one in." Ernest Hemingway, according to a bitchy Noel Coward lyric, could "just do it." Nunnally Johnson, the late and great Hollywood writer, once cabled a friend who had sailed off on a honeymoon with a bride thirty years younger, "You'll be all right—but don't show off."

Once you admit (to yourself and perhaps to her) you're no longer insatiable, you may both relax and surprise each other. If not, you will become a challenge, and women like challenges. Don't try too hard or her kisses may turn into mouth-to-mouth resuscitation. A man over fifty who tries to perform as though he were thirty had best wear a dog tag containing information as to blood type and next of kin. Another precaution is to use condoms, just as you did as a boy. They're ugly little things but they're for her protection too . . . against *your* sexual history.

After all this, you may be exhausted and reflect on how much safer it is to act your age in bed and adopt less strenuous means of gratification. But what are they?

My dear fellow, if you haven't learned by now how to satisfy a woman and yourself without an erection, you've been living in a tree. Books other than this one—or, preferably, a woman of experience—will teach you how, and you don't need appliances. Find a woman who has few inhibitions, no impossible performance expectations, and a passion for being touched. Try to be that way yourself. That kind of woman is sexy but nonchallenging. She was best described by the late George Jean Nathan as "someone who will not electrify me but with whom I can feel tenderly drowsy." He did find that someone in the beauteous Julie Haydon, and so can you find that someone. You don't want to be electrified. Who wants to be shocked—at your age?

You do have to be careful, especially if you are wed. Women have become so aggressive nowadays that you must sort out the possibles from the crazies. Remember the character Glenn Close played in the movie, *Fatal Attraction*? A crazy can ruin your life and send you screaming home to your wife, who may no longer want you. A crazy is someone who makes demands you can't or won't fulfill. They can be fiscal or sexual or social. You need to find someone whose needs are in harmony with yours. You must also be careful that you are with a discreet person. Any woman who regales you with tales of past loves (names included) obviously is to be avoided. The next name she mentions could be yours—and to someone who knows your wife.

Beware also of women who are all over you like a tent in a taxi or limousine—the overtly passionate kind. They are very seductive and it is flattering to find yourself the cause of so much heavy breathing, but I have found that these ladies cool off suddenly when they've snared you and tend to have rather nasty dispositions. Usually they're faking passion, as difficult as you may find that to believe.

My wife, Helen Gurley Brown, cautions older men to beware of the too young. They can age you quickly.

17

"Don't insist," she says, "on your women being younger than springtime—at least not *all* your women friends—or glossier than morning glory petals at dawn." Unless they have a father fixation, you're doomed to heartbreak. And besides, as Walter Matthau once said in a movie, "Who wants to go out with a girl who doesn't remember Ronald Colman?" Women closer to your own age know how to tend to your sexual hang-ups and will do so cheerfully, especially if you're single and available. They are more exciting in bed because they are more excitable and deprived, if not depraved. Their sexual prime is later than men's, which balances things nicely. No, it's not because older women are more grateful—that's a canard. They're more passionate than young women— and that's a fact.

In 1745 Benjamin Franklin wrote a friend advice on the choice of a mistress. This excerpt is worth quoting in full because it is as applicable today as it was two hundred and fifty years ago.

"In all your amours you should prefer old women to young ones . . .

"1. Because they have more knowledge of the world, and their minds are better stored with observations, their conversation is more improving and more lastingly agreeable.

"2. Because when women cease to be handsome they study to be good. To maintain their influence over men, they supply the dimunition of beauty by an augmentation of utility. They learn to do a thousand services great and small, and are the most tender and useful of friends when you are sick. Thus they continue amiable. And hence there is hardly such a thing to be found as an old woman who is not a good woman.

"3. Because there is no hazard of children, which irregularly produced may be attended with much inconvenience.

"4. Because through experience they are more prudent and discreet in conducting an intrigue to prevent suspicion. The commerce with them is therefore safer with regard to your reputation. And with regard to theirs, if the affair should happen to be known, considerate people might be rather inclined to excuse an old woman, who would kindly take care of a young man, form his manners by her good counsels, and prevent his ruining his health and fortune among mercenary prostitutes.

"5. Because in every animal that walks upright the deficiency of the fluids that fill the muscles appears first in the highest part. The face first grows lank and wrinkled; then the neck; then the breast and arms; the lower parts continuing to last as plump as ever; so that covering all above with a basket, and regarding only that which is below the girdle, it is impossible of two women to tell an old one from a young one. And as in the dark all cats are gray, the pleasure of corporal enjoyment with an old woman is at least equal, and frequently superior; every knack being, by practice, capable of improvement.

"6. Because the sin is less. The debauching a virgin may be her ruin, and make her life unhappy.

"7. Because the compunction is less. The having

made a young girl miserable may give you frequent bitter reflection; none of which can attend the making an old woman happy.

"8th and lastly. They are so gratefull."

While I find older women to be far better lovers, some men don't. The firm flesh, luminous eyes, and cascading hair of a nymphet can stir dangerous passions in an older man. She is the promise of renewed virility. Little wonder these men sometimes foresake family, fortune, and reason in their pursuit of the morning glory. Corporate states and empires have been reshaped by the young woman who has the old man in her thrall. Gene Fowler said, "One strand of pubic hair can be stronger than the Atlantic cable." You be stronger than your pubic hair.

If you're still not convinced, consider *your* appeal to a young woman. For openers, you're kidding yourself if you think she's mad for your body. (Older women will be.) I don't quite know who said it, but the words apply: "The love of an old man for a young woman is like sun on a mountaintop. It dazzles more than it warms." Also to the point, when asked about his love affairs with young girls, the motion-picture magnate Joseph Schenck, then in his seventies, said, "You can give a girl diamonds, sables, and Renoirs, but the time comes when she wants something substantial."

Now that we've straightened you out about the advisability, if not the desirability, of the older woman, how far do you go in this pursuit? Should you not wish the trouble, expense, and danger of an actual affair, there are, as I've mentioned earlier, less intimate but still tantalizing relationships to be had with other women—ones that will boost your ego and possibly extend your life span. Some of the most famous romantic liaisons have stopped short of the bedroom—have indeed been augmented by fantasies of what might have been. In literature (Tristan and Isolde) as well as in life (George Bernard Shaw and Mrs. Patrick Campbell) unconsummated relationships can be the headiest. Falling in love with someone who will never be yours is exquisitely poignant. The very impossibility of the relationship makes it obsessive. A long-ago, hidden romance of mine lost its spark when we both became free and able to see each other at will. We didn't, until we were safely married again—to others.

To get another woman in your life, flirt (cautiously, never blatantly)—at parties, in the office, on airplanes, in the supermarket. The world is filled with wonderful women who would like to know you—especially married women who may feel the same need as you do to keep relating to the opposite sex.

I'm always astonished by the frank, smiling looks of women I see on the streets, in buses or elevators—nice women, not hustlers. Engage in eye-lock with one or more of them and smile back. That may lead to a cup of coffee and perhaps something stronger later on. When you see one who seems to need you—and you'll be able to tell—ask her to lunch. Immediately find out what her problems are. Almost every love affair I've ever had started by my becoming either a confidant or a mentor (introducing her to those who could help her). You can win her trust by advising her about money or her difficulties at the office or at home. Ask *her* advice. She'll be flattered and it will bring her even closer.

Touch her. Women *like* to be touched if only on the elbow, hand, or shoulder to start. Holding hands while crossing the street comes naturally. You're not likely to be rebuffed. A kiss (lightly) on the lips will not be turned away. If you can manage to massage her neck on the pretext that she appears tense, you may have won her for life—no woman can resist a man's hands kneading her neck and drifting down to her shoulders and upper back. Of course, dancing is still the entry-level approach to intimacy, if you hold her delicately close with the promise of closer. "Women," wrote the British playwright Frederick Lonsdale, "crave appreciation more than anything else."

Having charmed and made a new friend, you can make arrangements for telephone calls. Relating to each other doesn't always mean an affair. Have lunch in well-known restaurants where you are *likely* to be seen. The choice of obscure places makes your relationship instantly obvious and somewhat shabby. Give small, thoughtful presents for Christmas and birthdays you can't spend with her. Avoid letters. Telephone instead—from booths or your office, of course.

As to how much you tell your mate about your new friend, that depends on your marital relationship. If it's a happy one and you don't make too much of these occasional lunches, she won't mind. Don't go into detail. Some of what you and your new friend talk about and do may not play well at home.

If something serious develops in your outside relationship, for heaven's sake don't ever confess. Observe again the sage words of playwright Lonsdale. "There are more men separated from their wives whom they love for that crime [telling the truth] than you and I would ever count. It's the most fatal thing in the world, believe me." I know a California couple who never wanted a divorce. One of them had strayed, and at the time the other felt that divorce was the only punishment that fit the crime. They saw each other later, and remarried. The straying one has now been forgiven but placed on permanent probation. They will live happily but warily forever after.

As for what you tell the other woman, the opposite applies. Never deceive her. She must know you are married and that your relationship with her will not escalate to that state (if you are bound to remain married). If she loves you and you are honest with her, she will remain with you—until *she* finds someone who will give her a more permanent relationship. If you're a sport, you'll give her away and nobody but she will be the wiser. While you are having your love affair, never cheat on her with still another woman—only with your wife. The real crimes of passion occur when the other woman discovers the other other woman. Murder and *merde!*

Romance late in life does have its price. Money, power, and fame are the aphrodisiacs that take the place of youthful virility and good looks. What, then, takes the place of marriage if you are already married and have no inclination or reason to split? Friendship, loving friendship. Men and women who are wed to others, make wonderful friends as well as lovers. Wives, even in the happiest alliances, rarely argue well (there are too many layers to the relationship), but a loving friend will let you win—occasionally. A man or woman can confide to a loving friend what he or she could not confide to a mate. In fact, a confidante is as good a remedy for depression as a therapist. Safe too. If she is the right one, she will die with your secrets even if you have parted in anger. A lady I loved kept my secret so well that after her death her sister, to whom she was very close, was astounded (and delighted) to hear—from me—of our love affair. My wife, upon learning that I would be late for dinner because of the funeral of this lady, grudgingly assented, "just as long as she's dead."

In an odd way life is enriched by having two loves. Almost everyone can love more than one person, but don't assume that if your mate dies your loving friendship will be better served by marriage. When playwright Ferenc Molnár's wife died, his friends, after a decent interval, suggested that now he could at last wed his mistress of long years. "But then," protested Molnár, "where would I spend my evenings?"

According to an article by Elton Duke titled "Franklin on Women" and published in *Old News*, "Whether a woman was young or old, lovely or homely, Franklin would go out of his way to flatter her and flirt. His flattery was based on genuine admiration. Franklin thought all women were wonderful, especially the clever ones."

Keep some love in *your* life, then—the bidden and forbidden—because love is the elixir of youth. An old Irish proverb holds, "Wherever you go, have a woman friend." Even a little flirtation triggers the adrenaline to flow. Whether girl-watching or the hard stuff, you will stay young all your life if you have a woman—preferably two of them, in case one falls out.

CHAPTER THREE

Marriage: Is It the Death of Romance?

I never met a girl I didn't marry. That's an exaggeration, of course (although I've been married three times), but it's no exaggeration to say I've never loved a girl I didn't want to marry or lusted after a girl I didn't think of marrying. All it took to make me horny (and eventually husbandly) was a pretty, preferably skinny, brunette in a black dress wearing a single strand of pearls. I guess that makes me the marrying kind.

Part of this passion for wedlock has to do with coming of age before the sexual revolution. When I was growing up, sex was still a big deal in America. You could tell a boy and girl were sleeping together when she ate something off his plate, but nobody went public with the relationship. The prevailing Puritanism begot hard-upness. Marriage was the only way to sleep with a desirable girl indefinitely. I didn't know that married girls could develop chronic headaches and that frigidity could occur in the summertime.

Life with the wrong mate can make Dante's Inferno seem like Disneyland. And yet, why is it that those caught in this hell often have to be routed out with flamethrowers? They seem to want to stay unhappy. One reason is you get used to the misery, the house, the car, the furniture, even her. It's scary and disorienting to leave home. You try to save the marriage, no matter what. My advice: Dump the marriage and save yourself.

Now that you're "saved," you must stay "saved." Another marriage is inevitable if your breath still registers in a mirror. Fine, but should you have children when you pass fifty? If you want to marry a young woman, she may insist. Some second families for older men provide much comfort and a feeling of renewed youth. Men often make better fathers the second time around. It can also be disastrous if you don't like children. It's better to have this issue settled before you become too involved. Tell her honestly how you feel.

Consider also that she may have more energy than you have. An article on middle-aged dating, in *The New York Times*, cautions older men to expect to have to go skiing when they would prefer to take a nap.

Still, don't marry someone closer to your age for companionship alone. She must be sexually interesting. A provocative female will make you feel and act young, even if she isn't. Sex is the down payment for any good man-woman relationship. Friendship and companionship are more likely to be based on good sex than common interests. As dwelled upon in the previous chapters (it *bears* repetition) there are lots of great-looking older women out there who are as rabbity as teenagers and also amusing and elegant. Grab one. She's looking for you. Treat her well. I repeat. Older women are more exciting than young ones and—surprise—sexually more demanding.

When I reflect upon my own marriage, I realize that a certain degree of tension and surprise is essential to continued interest in a mate. I never quite know what my wife will say or do, and although sometimes exasperating and even distressing, it keeps the relationship fresh and frisky. That's necessary if you're to avoid dead spells. Enid Bagnold once wrote, "Marriage: the beginning and the end are wonderful but the middle part is hell." It's interesting how well stormy marriages turn out if the partners stick together long enough.

Be careful about money in marriage. Think of the virtues of the somewhat stingy girl. Agreement about money is as vital as agreement about sex—and can affect sex. Her attitude about money reveals much of how she feels about you. Respect for money is respect for the one who is providing it. Hostility can drive a woman to spending orgies. It's a way of inflicting punishment.

Getting a credit rundown on a woman you're thinking of marrying isn't a bad idea. There's no reason why she shouldn't investigate your financial history too—whether she's worrying about your ability to support her or her need to support you.

If your wife has more money than you, your attitude toward her money may depend upon her attitude toward her money. Some rich women are exceedingly generous. They set up their poorer spouses with walking-around money, provide them with the great apartment, the country house, and even a place in the family business. Consequently, many older men who have been forced into retirement think life will be sweetened by marriage to a rich woman. Beware. This is traditionally the role of a prince consort, or conjugal "walker." A man must have a healthy ego or run the risk of losing his self-respect, particularly if after the marriage his wealthy wife starts to treat him as her possession. He had better know that a woman who buys him usually exacts a price. The price may be that he does exactly as she wishes. Nor can he depend upon getting her money if he's her willing creature. Most rich women I know are quite tight about money. Others demand prenup agreements and then require their husbands to assume the main support burden. And by the way, rich women can be killers when a marriage breaks up. They often demand and get more alimony than a poor woman, and they can afford the lawyers to prosecute and persecute.

Marriage to a woman more successful than you can work, provided you take pride in her achievements and are secure in your own. For years I was known as Helen Gurley Brown's husband, and frankly, I loved it. My peers knew who I was, but more importantly, I knew. Some women are comfortable with "weaker" men, and those marriages thrive, too, once the role of "house husband" is accepted.

Marriage is more than money and sex, although at the moment nothing else comes to mind. It's also about living together, which can be a problem if one's tastes and habits are wildly different. Every marriage has a secret contract with an unconditional-surrender clause. My wife would not consider separate bedrooms, for example. I sleep with her . . . gladly. If left alone, I would keep my radio on. I don't. Some might call this compromise. I call it surrender. My wife surrenders to my inability to throw out any scrap of paper including a dance card from a Stanford prom of 1934, and my predilection for untidy closets.

As for his and her friends, I've found it wise to tolerate her friends and relatives so that she will go easy on the ones I inflict on her. You don't have to drag her to parties you hate. You can make up an excuse for her—and she'll get you out of her animal rights dinner.

If she's a working girl, make her proud of you. Be a charmer, a true company husband. If one or both of you have to travel, don't fret. Separation can be good for the marriage. It adds zest and healthy yearning. Whatever you do on a business trip, don't tell your wife you did it, and pray she never confesses what she did. The flight attendant you took to dinner in Minneapolis is to remain unmentioned.

Is marriage the death of romance? It is easy to think so. Familiarity dulls the cutting edge. The strangeness of another female body, even if less attractive than your wife's, can flog a faltering libido into the danger zone. Monogamy does have its price. You may never know what it could be like with another woman, her style, her way, her laughter—but you can have your way with her in your fantasies and in your dreams.

What if you hear that your *wife* has had a real fling? If your marriage is solid—and you'll know if that's so—you'll give no credence to the rumor, although it will shake you up. I remember dancing with a friend of ours who insisted that my wife had had an affair with her husband. She wanted to make a lunch date so that "we could discuss what to do about it." As politely as I could, I extricated myself from both the dance and the lunch date. Years later I casually mentioned the incident to my wife but never asked whether what I had heard was true. Perhaps I didn't want to know. There *are* secrets even a husband and wife should not share. I advise you to let sleeping dogs lie—no matter whom they may be sleeping with.

CHAPTER FOUR

The Pains and Pleasures of Divorce

What little I know about marriage comes from knowing a good deal about divorce. I've been divorced twice. You would think it gets easier. It gets tougher. And yet the marital surgery that is divorce, I am convinced, saved my life. It may also have lengthened it.

A divorce sneaks up like a stranger in the night. You can feel it coming but you can't see it until it is upon you in the form of a lawyer's letter, a handwritten note at your breakfast plate, or a confrontation in the kitchen or bedroom in which the chilling words are uttered, "I want a divorce."

I'm writing this, of course, from a man's point of view. I've never asked for a divorce. I was always the divorced one, the limb that had to be sawed off, the one left in an empty home or dispatched to an impersonal hotel-room.

The knee-jerk reaction to a request for divorce—whether by wife or husband—is usually disbelief and a plea for time. A bad marriage must be preserved. That is what the partner who is being dumped, in desperation, wants. The dumper says she or he can't take it anymore and the dumpee promises to change, to buy extravagant gifts, and accept any conditions— but please don't leave. Someone I know sent a signed blank check to a departing wife, offering her everything to stay. A year later, he offered her everything to leave . . . having met his next wife.

It's hard to recall, years later, those awful feelings of being rejected; of being thrown out of a shared life, a home. However marred by disharmony, it is still a home. Without those familiar patterns of living one is left sadly disoriented. The immediate aftermath of a broken marriage, especially if there are children, is worse than the screaming fits and public embarrassments of a deteriorating relationship. You wake up at four in the morning and realize you're alone and a lot poorer. The only woman you want is the one you have lost.

Then, as subtly as the arrival of dawn, you begin to become aware of the outstretched arms waiting to enfold you. And they *will* be there, given the disheartening (to women) statistic that after fifty there are twenty men to every hundred women. As difficult as it may be to believe, an eligible sixty-year-old man can be the victim of gang rape.

Suddenly there are women for every need—women to tell you what an ungrateful wretch your ex-wife was; women to lend you money; women to invite you to their homes on Long Island or in the south of France; women to offer you chicken soup when you are ill and their bodies when you are well. Had I known this therapy for divorce existed, I would not have spent five years in psychoanalysis to discover how wonderful and deserving I was. Those women would have convinced me.

As tough as it is (at first) for a man to be dumped, it may be more agonizing for *him* to consider divorcing a faithful wife of many years. The subject of breaking up may never have arisen, even though he has been stuck in a loveless, sexless, humorless relationship. The fires of passion have long since turned to ashes, and he's the one who has had to carry out the ashes. Does he *dare* ask for a divorce at this stage of their lives? She is probably over fifty now (remember there are a hundred of her age to every twenty of his age). The children are no doubt grown and gone. In her role as full-time wife and mother, she has not acquired any skills to serve her in the job market. As for another man, forget it. Can he throw her to the wolves when there are no wolves?

The answer is he can, but not without a large measure of guilt. He will find a new wife, but chances are she is being cast into a manless void. Saving himself may seem selfish, and it is—but he can't save her or the marriage by remaining. Children are no longer an issue. They're usually gone by now. My advice to him is to get out, too, as speedily as he got into the marriage, and suffer the guilts.

One of the sad realities of divorce is that the divorced ones rarely remain friends. It's war. He (or she) who has been left is generally considered the victim. The woman will have the harder time, but if she hones her sexual skills as well as her body and *likes* men, there is a chance, albeit a slim one, of making a good second marriage.

Money is the ruling passion of divorce, and also the ultimate weapon. Consequently, the price of freedom comes high, especially if there is another woman. For an affluent defector the severance package can be as complex and as rich as that of a departing executive of a multinational corporation. Big or small, a settlement, or alimony award, will be fraught with bitterness. When I was summoned into the presence of Louis Nizer, the famed attorney who represented my first wife, I uttered words that were to impoverish me for years: "Show me where to sign." The cost seemed of no consequence, but later each payment enraged and sickened me. Fortunately, she remarried and I was soon released from paying alimony. My second wife, having observed my reaction to my first wife's demands, mercifully asked nothing when *she* left.

I've concluded, somewhat reluctantly, that it is better to pay the price of the divorce with as little rancor and inconvenience as possible and get on with your life.

As for your future relationship with your ex, much depends upon the circumstances of your departure or hers. If you are remarried to a woman half her age (and yours), don't expect flowers on your birthday. I've found it is best to stay away from ex-wives unless there are child-custody requirements that bring you together. If you do not have a woman in your life and your ex has not remarried, it may be dangerous to see her, especially if one of you still has a "thing" for the other. I once took my first ex-wife to the theater (I don't remember why) and back to her apartment and felt an urge to bed her. There is something libidinous and deliciously forbidden about a still beautiful ex. In some courts resumption of sexual relations cancels a legal separation. Stay away unless you don't mind remarrying her. What hooked you in the first place may rehook you.

If you are the victim of the vengeance of an angry ex-wife, you may be harassed to your grave if you don't take countermeasures. You may have to start a new life elsewhere. A better defense may be a tough new wife. Nobody can put down an old wife as fearlessly as a new wife. Your old wife has your number. Not just your telephone number but the ability to arouse you to incredible fury with some trivial complaint, and your overreaction will bring her inexpressible pleasure. She knows *that*. When my old wife telephoned, my lower back would turn to cement—on which she was chiseling expletives. A new wife will have no such emotional reaction and can tell your former wife to buzz off. The old wife will soon get over the fun of riling you up and perhaps go away.

Old wives don't die if they're getting alimony, and rarely remarry unless they find someone richer than you. They do fade away, however, and leave you wondering what the *Sturm und Drang* was all about. Eventually, it will seem as though it all happened to someone else. As for the alimony you pay, the rationale may lie in a Broadway cynic's definition of that hated tribute: "Alimony is the screwing you get for the screwing you got."

For those who, for religious reasons, cannot contemplate divorce, separation or annulment may be the only remedy. I think it's ungodly to perpetuate a cruel relationship. Surely, a merciful deity never intended anyone to withstand verbal or physical abuse, drug or alcoholic madness, banishment from the marriage bed.

War is hell, but divorce is worse—at first. Later, it may turn out to be one of the best things you've ever done. Even if you haven't met the right woman (and she may be looking for you this very moment), you have the peace and quiet of an untroubled relationship—with yourself.

CHAPTER FIVE

The Care and Feeding of the Older Body

After seventy, if you wake up without pains, you're dead, observed a friend of literary critic Malcolm Cowley, himself at the time a presumably pain-racked eighty-nine. Long before seventy, however, you become aware that things are not what they were. You can't run as fast. Tennis singles turn into doubles. You begin to lose your way a little, and you forget things. Young women no longer give you the Look, and, horrors, a pregnant lady gives you a seat on the bus.

It gets worse.

You will notice, perhaps for the first time, that many, and then most, of those around you are younger.

By fifty there are changes in your hairline and your hair color. One consolation is that you probably won't lose any more hair than you have already; but, unless you're Ronald Reagan, your hair will turn gray and then white.

Those feats of sexual power—making it two or three times a night—will dwindle to a precious few and you'll be grateful for them, as will she. After too few years the Big O had become the Big Ordeal. Old faithful . . . or unfaithful, as may be the case . . . cannot be relied upon to rise on cue.

Late night clubs will no longer seem the place to be—too noisy, too jumpy. Worse, you may think they're too quiet. Some loss of hearing can occur as early as one's mid-fifties, and you will also have to accommodate yourself to poorer eyesight. No longer can you read a paperback book in a tunnel. When you give in to wearing glasses, don't complain that you have become dependent upon them. You have. I put on my glasses when I answer the telephone.

The one thing you will do more of is go to the bathroom. Your plumbing system is aging and as prone to leaks and stoppages as the New York water system. I know the location of every men's room, and in fact, I can draw a map of their whereabouts in all major hotels, theaters, restaurants, and museums in the principal cities of the world, including a neat little facility in the Gobi Desert.

Gruesome, isn't it?

Soon you will become aware that quite a number of your friends have suffered serious illnesses, and not a few have died. You will start reading the obituary pages before the sports pages. Interestingly you will be aware of the imminence of death.

Barring accidents, whether you die now or later may depend on how well you care for your body.

Good health is beautifully boring. You don't even

think about it while you have it. Illness is not. Your objective should be to remain healthfully bored. Can doctors help?

Admittedly eccentric, I have long suspected that seeing a physician when you are feeling fit can be dangerous. What if he "finds" something that isn't there? Phenomenally successful movie and record producer David Geffen dropped out of the entertainment business for three years, believing he was dying of cancer. He wasn't. The diagnosis was wrong. Investment banker William Salomon required a hip operation and took the precaution of painting with iodine the side on which he was to be operated. He was not paranoid. Actress Peggy Cass came out of surgery to discover that the wrong knee had been operated on. Motion picture executive Taft Schreiber, a benefactor of a California hospital, died following a transfusion during a minor operation. Reportedly, a medical clerk had mislabeled a bottle of blood.

Andrew Stein, president of the New York City Council, once wrote, "The Ralph Nader organization's Health Research group estimates that as many as 200,000 Americans are injured or killed in hospitals each year as a result of negligent care. . . . Dr. Arnold Reiman, editor of *The New England Journal of Medicine*, believes that at least 20,000 grossly incompetent or negligent doctors continue to practice in this country—and that the figure may in fact be twice as high." In the June 1986 issue, the twenty-eight million readers of *Reader's Digest* learned a new word: *iatrogenic*. It means any illness that is "doctor induced."

On a recent flight from New York to Los Angeles, a Nobel Prize-winning medical researcher at the University of California was seated next to me. In the course of a five-hour conversation he begged me never to accept the recommendation of a single physician, especially when it related to surgery. He urged me—loudly—to get a second, third, or even fourth opinion. I did, fortunately, for my (blessed) prostate operation.

What he was saying was that doctors are not necessarily gods. When I was a young man, I worked as a lobbyist for the American Medical Association. Our headquarters in Chicago was filled with M.D.'s in high administrative jobs. A fair number of them, I believe, would have fainted at the sight of blood, and I would not have trusted any of them to apply a Band-Aid. When someone you haven't checked out tells you he's practicing medicine, he may indeed only be practicing . . . one hopes not on you.

Such doctors are, happily, in the minority. Many more *are* godlike, caring and unmotivated by greed. Shop around for one. Ask friends. Check the county medical society for accreditations. At some time in your life, his or her skills will be crucial to you. There are no doctor-doubters in operating rooms, and if you find the right M.D., you needn't be one of the appalling statistics I have cited. However, you must bear the responsibility of *selecting* the right doctor.

One way I benefit from medical advice is occasionally to take heed of what doctors have advised friends to do. An example: Some years ago a motion picture producer I knew had a heart attack and nearly died. After his recovery I asked him what had been prescribed for the prevention of another heart attack and took notes while he revealed his new diet. After we had returned home, I told my wife that I was going to pretend that I had had a heart attack and adopt the same regimen as my stricken friend had. I followed the same diet my friend was on, took off fifty pounds, and have survived twenty years beyond his death (and he was younger than I).

The medical profession may condemn me for suggesting that you can be your own best doctor at times. Yet old friend H. B. Brown, Jr., had to be his own doctor. He was badly shaken up in an automobile accident, which left him with almost permanent pain in his back. His doctors told him that he could choose either to live with the pain or have an operation, but gave no assurance that the operation would be a success. Faced with these odds, H. B. had no alternative except to live with it and suffer. He had heard that one way to relieve back pain is to breathe deeply, but the problem was he had great difficulty breathing. One day he read that in certain areas of Europe beekeepers live to be well past a hundred and that, to breathe more easily, these beekeepers ingested bee pollen, or the residue left over when they sold the honey. H. B. found some in a health store and gradually increased the dosage until he could breathe freely. His back soon stopped aching. He's still on the bee pollen and is now well and a robust eighty-three.

You can be your own doctor regarding alcohol— I've found too many physicians are noncommittal about its use. As early as your late forties you will notice a lessening of your ability to consume alcohol, sometimes after only two drinks. Your voice will slur and though your brain seems as nimble as ever, the words don't come out sharp and clear. You try to fake it by speaking slowly and overenunciating, but a keen ear will not be deceived.

That's a good reason to consider cutting down. Going without alcohol for even a week will make you feel better than you ever imagined you could. My friend Ambassador Franklin S. Forsberg is a man who seems never to have aged, although he is now over eighty. Frank enjoys a drink at lunch, but for one month each year he abstains completely—nothing and nobody can make him take a drink. He uses that dry month to get his system back in balance and lose a few pounds.

Frank is a good drinker. There are not many of those. While some studies show that moderate consumption of alcohol can reduce the risk of heart attacks up to fifty percent, there are other risks.

I have found that even a small amount of alcohol can also change your personality. You may be fooled because you don't sound all that different to yourself, but others will notice you're saying things that are unlike you, things that may anger and sadden those dear to you.

I've come closest to wrecking my marriage and friendships while drinking, even moderately. Drinking often releases sudden and inexplicable combativeness, repressed aggressions and paranoia.

When I contemplated writing this book, I vowed I would come out in favor of wine and whiskey and other alcoholic drinks. I do like to drink a little. Nothing is quite so euphoric, for example, as that first drink on an airplane when the stress of takeoff is behind you and you are comfortably airborne. I can't imagine a decent meal without a drink, although whiskey dulls the palate and is frowned upon in really first-class restaurants. My message, then, is to cut down (and not out) and to avoid all alcoholic beverages in situations where there is apt to be pressure or tension, or when you are fatigued. In other words, unless you're an alcoholic and can't drink at all, drink moderately when happy but not at all when tired, tense, or angry. On guard!

For a sterner regimen to remain astonishingly youthful (as he has in his seventies) Mike Abrums, the health guru to Hollywood's high and mighty, has five "no-no's." You will observe from the previous paragraph that I do not agree with the first commandment of Mike Abrums but here are his "no-no's":

No booze
No salt
No sugar
No fat
No red meat

To which I am tempted to add a sixth "no"—"no fun."

I'm not keen about exercise. If it pleases you and makes you feel good, do it. A Stanford study states that losing weight only by dieting is as effective in reducing cholesterol and blood pressure as exercise alone.

My friend Virginia Salomon chooses strenuous exercise. She swims sixty-two laps each morning. I asked whether it made her feel wonderful. "Terrible," she exclaimed. "Not swimming makes me feel wonderful." Dr. Christian Barnard agrees. "Exercise is like a cold bath," says Barnard. "You feel better after you finish with it."

There is no medical evidence that exercise extends life and there are some doctors who believe it shortens it. I'm referring to the kind of exercise that puts sweat on a middle-aged body and makes the heart pump like an oil drill. Tennis is fine if you're in good shape already—golf is harmless and probably beneficial. Walking and swimming are best, I've found, and it's not boring if you walk with someone agreeable, preferably a dog. As for swimming, that is the swiftest way to reap the benefits of exercise. A ten-minute swim every other day is all you need. Dr. Laurence E. Morehouse and Leonard Gross, in their book *Total Fitness in Thirty Minutes a Week*, say ten minutes of peak effort every day will earn eighty percent of the cardiovascular-conditioning benefits of hours of exercise every day. Read their book to find out what's *peak* for you.

Most recent studies, according to an article by health expert Jane Brody, indicate strongly that *moderate* exercise late in life reverses many of the effects of aging. Such exercise is beneficial no matter when you start or how out of shape you are. If you start early enough, according to these studies, you can set back your biological clock as much as twenty-five to forty-five years. Moreover, the article states, "You don't have to run marathons to reap the benefits. For the average older person who does little more than rapid walking for thirty minutes at a time three or four times a week, it can provide ten years of rejuvenation."

The quest for longer life reportedly led such power figures as Pope Pius XII, former German Chancellor Konrad Adenauer, and Sir Winston Churchill to have transplants of fetal lamb cells. They all did live long. Nobel laureate Linus Pauling avowed that megadoses of vitamin C would extend life sixteen to twenty-four years and keep you fit besides. H. L. Hunt used to creep on all fours several times a day to keep fit, and Adenauer, fetal lamb cells and all, believed standing erect would fight off infirmities. He died at ninety-one.

A gerontologist at Rockefeller University, who would prefer his name not to be mentioned, says the Three Commandments for a long, healthy life are: (1) eat half of what you do now; (2) exercise regularly; (3) have sex every day.

As for his first commandment, experiments with mice at Cornell University as early as 1935 proved that underfed mice lived fifty percent longer than mice who were fed as much as they wanted. Dr. Roy Walford of the UCLA School of Medicine repeated the experiment in the seventies and found that whenever the undernutrition started, the animals still lived a third longer than the overfed ones. Most of the men and women I know who have reached the age of eighty or more are thin. George Delacorte, Jr., in his nineties, still walked several miles a day, but ate like a leprechaun. John Loeb, the venerable New York banker, is ninety-one and as skinny as a man can be and still keep a good tailor. He was given only a forty-percent change of living when he contracted cancer in his thirties—but look at him now! Irving Berlin, at ninety-nine, didn't weigh much more than his age.

It's up to you. Some may not call it living to take in fifteen hundred calories a day as Dr. Walford does (applying his mice experiment to himself). In this case, please ask your doctor before you start starving yourself, preferably a doctor who knows nutrition.

You *can* be too thin. Some of my older friends, particularly from California, appear to be hastening the process of skeletonization. That will come. Now that they can afford a good meal, they look as though they've been released from Intensive Care. I agree women can't be too thin. Skinny women look younger, but skinny men look mummified.

Don't take this as a plea for fatness—merely an appeal for rational dieting. Eat just enough to fill out those facial wrinkles. Don't go on an all-protein, non-sugar diet. I tried this and became so irritable that

47

nobody would talk to me. The body craves carbohydrates, and a *little* sugar will make up for a lot of alcohol. I eat sparingly of red meats but fill up on leafy vegetables (cabbage, brussels sprouts), which may be cancer deterrents. Whatever fruits and vegetables are in season should be eaten then, before chemicals and preservatives have been added. Nutrition experts advise taking twenty-five to thirty-five grams of fiber each day and can tell you the best natural sources. Decaffeinated coffee may not taste as good, but you avoid that hyped-up feeling. Yukiko Irwin (about whom more later), drawing on the wisdom of her ancestor, Ben Franklin (himself a health nut), as well as Confucius, urges saintly moderation in all things (eating, sex on which, as noted, Ben and she part company—and other pleasures) and dwelling on the positive in your thoughts.

As for vitamins (particularly tryptophan, vitamin E, and vitamin C), I regard them the same way as I do religion. I take them because their adherents may be right—just as I worship because I don't want to be left out if the religionists are right.

Linus Pauling was one of those "religionists." He once wrote: "I believe if people were to avoid sucrose—hardly ever spoon out a spoonful of sugar from the sugar bowl onto anything, avoid sweet desserts except when you're a guest somewhere, avoid buying foods that say 'sugar' as one of the contents—they would cut down on the incidence of disease and increase life expectancy. Take a fair amount of vitamins. Stop smoking cigarettes. And you'll have a longer and happier life—more vim and vigor and a better time altogether." Pauling believes a one-pack-a-day smoker had twice as much chance of dying of heart disease as a nonsmoker, and a two-pack-a-day smoker had four times as much chance. He also stated, "With the proper use of ascorbic acid (vitamin C), the mortality from cancer might well be decreased by fifty percent."

For Erté, the eminent fashion designer, illustrator, and sculptor, work was the best way to care for the older body. At ninety-five he was as busy as he was in the nineteen twenties. "I don't need drugs to go away," he commented in an interview in the *San Francisco Examiner*, "because when I'm working, I'm on another planet."

For leisurely hours, an obvious tip. The sun ages the skin, makes you look older, can even lead to skin cancer. I stay out of it, never having subscribed to Aristotle Onassis' dictum "Always have a tan in winter." I prefer Noel Coward's observation "Mad dogs and Englishmen go out in the noonday sun."

Cigarette smoking may be pleasurable for some but lethal, if not illegal, for most. I smoke cigars, but only the finest Havanas. The aroma is fragrant and a cigar complements a superb dinner. I smoke only one or two a day, and never in public. My wife does not complain. When I decided to marry her, I did not ask whether she loved me but whether she loved cigars. She was wise enough to say yes—and in thirty-two years has never reneged. The only criticism of pipe smokers I have heard came not from the Surgeon

General but from Jack Warner, the late movie mogul. Warner said, "Beware of a man who smokes a pipe. He may be thinking."

Massages are magical, particularly the Japanese shiatsu kind. They keep the blood flowing and break up potential clots. My therapist, Yukiko Irwin, is a miracle worker and is regularly referred patients by renowned New York physicians.

I have found it untrue that the older you get the less sleep you need. Observe an older cat or dog dozing off at frequent intervals. That's you. To confuse matters, you are also likely to suffer from insomnia. The syndrome is common. After two or three hours of deep sleep you are as awake as a hungry leopard. Avoid sleeping pills, even the milder nonbarbiturate variety. They can be scarily disorienting with Alzheimer-like effect. Instead, get up and start answering letters; read Tolstoy or Toynbee. Prepare hot tea. If none of these works, count the women you've loved instead of counting sheep; relive your childhood by threading up the past and playing it in the theater of your mind. Sing popular songs in your head. You will never be off pitch. Remembering the lyrics will be a soporific.

Stay calm and don't overreact to petty crises. They're the worst. For an elaboration on this theme read *Is It Worth Dying For?* by Dr. Robert S. Eliot and Dennis L. Breo.

Simply don't try to win every argument. Lose some. Winning may shorten your life. It's not necessary always to be on time, or flagellate yourself when you are late. May Robson, active in films into her eighties, described her secret of endurance as "not rushing." Don't try to see everything or everybody. In Noel Coward's later years he observed, "People are always telling me about something I have just missed. I find it very restful." Reduce stress by diminishing expectations. Accept the limits. In Rio de Janerio the Cariocas say, "If you miss the plane, you can go back to the hotel, have a drink, and relax—so there's no problem. If you make the plane, there's no problem." Perhaps you ought to let a little Brazil into your life. Be loose. Do your best but not your utmost. You will achieve more by cultivating serenity and poise. Pace yourself by accepting the limits and thereby making do with less stress and tension.

I'm against "overdoctoring," but you may not have filled out a medical history and reminded yourself of what your parents died from—and at what ages. One good reason to see a doctor is to monitor your body for ailments that may be hereditary. However you find out, it is a good idea to avoid whatever brings on the serious illnesses your parents had. Example: if diabetes was a cause of death, skip the sugar. If lung cancer ended a parent's life, stop smoking. If pushing himself too hard did your father in, slow down. If your mother worried herself to death (mine did), relax.

I'm not suggesting that growing older is wonderful. Shakespeare's *King Lear* is a devastating portrait of the erosion of body and spirit that aging produces. And yet, nothing can outweigh the wonder of still being here. And as for the limits, they need not be a depressant. You've had your "limitless" years. The Chinese philosopher Lao Tzu wrote, "Things become old through an excess of vigor." Be grateful some of your vigor survived. That's why, for you, the party goes on even though many who arrived with you have had to leave early.

You can be healthy almost to the hour of death. Actress Ruth Gordon was, when she died in her sleep at eighty-eight. Ultimately, the body must fail—but how much better to fail all at once so that your dying words will make sense.

CHAPTER SIX

It's Not Over till
It's Over

"Like children falling asleep over their toys," intoned the rabbi at a service for Senator Jacob K. Javits, "we relinquish our grasp on earthly possessions only after death overtakes us. . . ."

Death is a spoilsport. Just when you're wise enough to know how to play, it comes along and breaks up the game. About the only ones who welcome the intruder are those for whom life is more painful than the anticipation of death. Try to find one. Intensive-care wards are jammed with people fighting to stay alive, tubes and paraphernalia coming out of every vein and orifice. Denial of death is a deception practiced from birth onward. People—especially "important" people—act as if they never expect to die, confirming what Woody Allen says in his life-affirming movie *Hannah and Her Sisters*, that if we really believed death was inevitable it would spoil everything in between. And yet we *are* all under sentence of death, even though the sentence may be suspended; as Thomas Gray wrote in his "Elegy in a Country

Churchyard," ". . . all that beauty, all that wealth e'er gave,/Awaits alike th' inevitable hour:/The paths of glory lead but to the grave."

Whenever it occurs, rationally, we ought not to fear death. William Hazlitt, who may now have experienced the truth of his words, observed, "There was a time when we were not; this gives us no concern— why, then, should it trouble us that a time will come when we shall cease to be?"

Why, indeed? Oblivion or whatever, I am still troubled by the contemplation of being separated eternally from my wife, friends, work, occasional grand passions, and certain restaurants in New York, Paris, London, and Lyon. Quite apart from these earthly pleasures, I don't want to leave my bed for some damp, untended grave, there to repose forever under snow and rain and the light of distant stars.

It's unbelievable—from its abruptness to the look of it. In an instant life is over—the memories, the lusts, the hopes, the fantasies. In death the contorted bodies seem more like broken mannequins. Only the eyes, if not closed, are real—staring at what we shall have to wait to see.

But what if, as some religions hold, we are not consigned to a void after death? According to a *New York Times* report, more than eight million people have had "near-death" experiences, in which many say "that they enter a tunnel of darkness and move towards a brilliant white light which emits warmth and love, that they are flooded with knowledge beyond their ordinary capabilities, that they discover the pattern or meaning of life." One caution. We may also find ex-wives and former enemies whom we were pleased to have precede us. Depending on the makeup of the celestial welcoming committee, we may not know whether we're in heaven or hell.

And if reincarnation is our fate, and we are to return in a different persona, what assurances do we have that we will not be exchanging a seat on the New York Stock Exchange for one behind an oar on the River Ganges? My idea of heaven is spending one's next life with an old love even if our past life together is beyond recall. How would I know her? Lyricist Lorenz Hart put it poignantly when he wrote:

> *Some things that happen for the first time*
> *Seem to be happening again.*
> *And so it seems that we have met before,*
> *And laughed before, and loved before,*
> *But who knows where or when?*

For those of us who fear death, perhaps the easiest course is to fight it. Dylan Thomas exhorts: "Do not go gentle into that good night,/Old age should burn and rave at close of day;/Rage, rage against the dying of the light." If you are not up to a fight, consider this gentler plea from beyond by an unknown (to me) poet.

> Do not stare at my grave and weep.
> I am not there. I do not sleep.

I am a thousand winds that blow.
I am the diamond glints on snow.
I am the sunlight on ripened grain.
I am the gentle autumn rain.
When you awaken in the morning's hush,
   I am the swift uplifting rush.
of quiet birds in circled flight.
   I am the soft stars that shine at night.
Do not stand at my grave and cry.
   I am not there. I did not die.

Whether you "rage," or resign yourself to the inevitable, don't waste time brooding over those days of lengthening shadows.

Live riotously. It is foolish to sit around waiting for the collector when the collector may be late. Baseball coach Yogi Berra taught us that "it's not over till it's over." And if Larry Hart, the New Testament, Buddha, and the Koran are right, it may not be over even then. You'll either be with your pals in paradise or you won't feel a thing.

CHAPTER SEVEN

What Is Success, Anyhow?

Sometime in life—it may be as early as your fortieth birthday—you may ask yourself whether you have succeeded or failed in life. Or you may block out the question altogether. A realization will sweep over you that this is it. Whatever you were going to become, you've become. You wanted more. You mourn the death of youthful hopes. Dumb, dumb, dumb. How could you have blown it?

Or, sometime in life—it may be as late as your eightieth birthday—you celebrate your luck, which by now you have rationalized as talent and wisdom. While others were failing all around you, you, dear boy, made those millions, or became famous, or both. You look admiringly upon your young wife, for whom you traded in your old one. She was worth the cost. All of it was. Now all you have to do is stay alive.

Later life is settlement time for all you've done or failed to do in earlier years. If you've abused your body, you are a wreck at fifty, gaga at sixty, and facing a too-early but welcome death. If you've wasted twenty adult years in pointless but pleasing foolery, you pay by becoming unemployable and not being able to pay your bills. You are an embarrassment. Poverty is becoming only to the young and promising. If, conversely, you have obsessively and single-mindedly pursued success, fame, riches—whether in commerce or the arts—you may pay by not having the time to enjoy yourself, or having so narrow a range of interests as to make you a bore.

None of the above constitutes success. Fulfilling youthful goals does not make one successful. The goals may be wrong. Being unable to measure up to talk-show standards of success—i.e., wealth, celebrity, or notoriety—is not failure. Success itself is not a constant. You may think yourself a success at forty and a failure at sixty. It comes and goes and often ruins the recipient in its passage. The author Scott Fitzgerald said, "Nothing fails like success." His sad life proved it. My friend Herbert R. Mayes added "Nothing recedes like success." Too true. Marilyn Monroe pensively wrote, "Good-bye fame. I've had you, fame." Hers was not a successful life.

Once lost, conventional success leads one into darker pits of despair than is ever experienced by those who have never made it to the top. Stephen Sondheim wirtes a loser's lament in one of his memorable lyrics from *Follies*:

> *Success is swell*
> *And success is sweet,*
> *But every height has a drop.*
> *The less achievement,*
> *The less defeat.*

What Is Success, Anyhow?

What's the point of shovin'
Your way to the top?

Even when success stays around, there is that ogre about whom Nietzsche wrote when he observed that each desire fulfilled leads to new ones that demand fulfillment. It isn't enough to achieve success. One must dwarf it by greater subsequent achievements. The late David O. Selznick, not content with having produced the screen's greatest masterpiece, *Gone With the Wind*, spent the rest of his life immobilized by his triumph. He would never find another subject that, in his view, would remotely equal his earlier triumph. My wife, ordinarily a modest and realistic person, swore that if she could see one of her books listed for *one* week on the *New York Times* Best Seller List she would forever be content. She wasn't. Her books remained on the *New York Times* Best Seller List for months, but the week they dropped off it was as though there had been a death in the family.

Irving Berlin summarized the situation when he remarked, "The toughest thing about success is that you have to keep on being a success."

I think success is not so much doing what you want as wanting what you do. If you make a fortune working at something you hate or are ashamed of, you have failed. Johnny Carson once advised, "Never continue in a job you don't enjoy. If you're happy in what you're doing, you'll like yourself; you'll have inner peace. And if you have that, along with physical health, you will have had more success than you could possibly have imagined."

Success is most satisfying when you have someone you love to share it with. If you make other persons realize *their* potential, you will know special joy. Many successful persons feel guilty because they are so much better off than most of mankind. They help others, often anonymously. One of my good and rich friends identifies some especially needy and worthy person or family and does something that will help them materially. His only condition is that his name never be revealed. Frank Sinatra is another whose anonymous gifts are numerous and substantial, in addition to his public philanthropy. These are successful persons.

Real success cannot be achieved without integrity and adherence to moral values. This may seem anachronistic in a society where the Golden Calf is worshiped and, in Cole Porter's words, "anything goes." To achieve wealth by "dirty tricks," dishonesty, or ruthlessness won't buy you the respect of your family or peers. They almost always know what you are. Walter Winchell was one of the most powerful men of his time. Kings and presidents read his newspaper column. Stocks rose when he mentioned a company favorably. He wrote in his column, "Be nice to the people you meet on the way up. They're the same ones you see on the way down." Evidently, he wasn't. He used his power to destroy those who crossed him. The only people at his funeral were paid to be there.

Success is a man whose children love him and have made him proud of them. My friend Gene Shalit is such a man. Famous as a critic and television personality, he considers his greatest achievement the love and respect of his six children, who are themselves highly gifted. Through the illness and following the death of their mother he had full responsibility for their upbringing. He motivated them to care for one another and be self-reliant, but the pressures of his network job never kept him from being available. When they went away to school, each child was given a telephone credit card with no limitation as to the number of calls as long as they called one another. Not one child violated this condition.

Success is a man who has the love and trust of a woman, a job he likes and excels at, and an abiding sense of humor.

Success is someone who has written a concerto or a novel that he believes is his best work—never mind the critics or the sales. It is also an actor who on one night of a three-year run of a play has given a performance that was so pure he thought it must have come from someone else. Success was Yul Brynner. It is also Woody Allen.

Success is a man who does his job superbly and has total control of his life and work. Such a man is Marten Cornelissen, who emigrated from Holland to Northampton, Massachusetts, where he makes violins and violas in a house as unimposing as the one in which Stradivari lived and worked in Italy. They say Cornelissen's instruments may be as good as Stradivari's when they ripen in a century or two. Right now they are very good.

Success is a man who dies at home in his sleep after a good life.

Success is what makes you and others feel good. Anything that makes you or others feel bad, regardless of the money you make, is failure.

Honest failure, the inability to live up to one's expectations, is mixed up with success. Most living is at least three parts failure to one part success. Nothing works perfectly and nobody has it all. In order to succeed, one must risk and endure failure. As with success, failure comes and goes. It is not constant unless you stop trying. Merely working at something good that doesn't quite come off is a kind of success—if the work is good.

I will not be hypocritical and say that money and power are not pleasing. I agree with Sophie Tucker's quip, "I've been poor and I've been rich and rich is better." But then, why do I know so many miserable rich people? Perhaps because they obtained their riches in a miserable way—and they know it.

Sybaritic pleasures are worth their prices to those who have made a study of good living. For me, fine wines, French haute cuisine, and cigars from Havana (Churchill size) are what I would hope to find in heaven. Surely smoking is permitted in some distant corner up there (where nothing is hazardous to your health)—or what's a heaven for? I pity those who have achieved affluence but lack the taste to enjoy it. Malcolm Forbes knew how to live beautifully and generously. So did W. R. Hearst. And yet one needn't be rich to know the rare delights the world offers. In my youth I spent more on fine cigars and wine than on rent.

There are, of course, other measures of achievement. Success is being determined to stay alive and do something with the rest of your life. I urge you to spend your later years either in trying to remain successful, as Irving Berlin put it, or reversing your failures by trying again.

As for envy, forget it. Study the words of Alexander Solzhenitsyn. "If your back isn't broken, if your feet can walk, if both arms can bend, if both eyes can see, and if both ears hear, then whom should you envy? And why? Our envy of others devours us most of all. Rub your eyes and purify your heart and prize above all else in the world those who love you and who wish you well."

That's success.

CHAPTER EIGHT

Tyranny of the Practical

Actually, if I did have another life I might prefer to come back as a plasterer, plumber, or electrician. For the lack of a plumber an otherwise happy family can be turned into a snake pit of frustration. Awards, success, money, health, become meaningless while you await helplessly the arrival of the man who can stop the water pipes from hemorrhaging into your state-of-the-art personal computer while also trickling onto your one decent painting.

My old friend the late Milton Gordon had devised a neat trick that enabled him to attract all the workmen he needed and at once. He let it be known that he didn't mind being cheated. Upon receipt of the first exorbitant bill for some trifling job, he telephoned the roofer, electrician, or whomever and exlaimed, "I received your bill and it's a relief to find how reasonable it is." After this call, plasterers, tile men, electricians, and plumbers lined up to work for Milton while neighbors went into cardiac arrest because they couldn't get anyone to fix anything in their lifetime. It was worth the overcharge, said Milton.

Art Buchwald has a clever scheme to ensure that

workmen keep their appointments. He knows where they hang out at breakfast and goes there to make sure his man does not tarry or get lost on his way to the Buchwalds'. He has even been known to pick up a breakfast tab to hurry his man on his way to work.

You might think billionaire Robert Tisch, whose hotel empire employs skilled craftsmen all over the world, could get a workman to his apartment on demand and a break on price. Not so, a friend of his told me. Mr. Tisch, who carefully scrutinizes labor costs at his office, rarely questions repair bills for his home. His time is worth more than the psychic cost of futile bickering.

For those who are less inclined to be generous, or can't get up early enough to meet the plumber for breakfast, there are other means. Whatever needs repairing may not need repairing—yet. Live with it. You may live longer that way than enduring the torture of trying (and failing) to get it fixed. A dripping faucet can go on dripping for years without causing damage. Let it drip.

Another thought. Try to discover your tradesman's secret ambition in life. If he wants to be an actor, ask a producer friend to give him a reading. Maybe he wants to write. Encourage him to let you read his coffee-stained manuscript. His daughter may yearn to be a model. Ask a photographer friend to take pictures of her. Keep your man's hopes high and you'll never suffer a broken appointment to fix a broken pipe. You can string him along for years while your home remains in perfect repair.

Never pay any portion of a bill in advance. Work tends to be completed more rapidly when money is owed. Leave liquor around and available, especially for house painters. Whether they mix it with the paint or not, it tends to get used up and the job proceeds faster. If you hide the booze, time is wasted until they find it (and find it they will).

Let each of your key workmen know he's on your Christmas list and remind him the list is incomplete when you need a job done in November. For your most important workmen, tell them they're in your will and occasionally act faint and stagger a bit.

Don't pick a fight with a tradesman. It is better to let your wife walk out than have a roofer leave in anger. You can get a new wife but may never get another roofer . . . or any other workman. Word gets out that you're hard to please. Another reason not to fight these chaps is that they can kill you with one of their tools and claim self-defense.

Some appliances can be fixed by dropping them. A toaster, for example. Don't drop a television set, however. They tend to explode. Unless you're a mechanical genius, fixing them yourself can be dangerous. A friend of mine attempted to repair an electrical connection, with the result that astonished neighbors observed sheet lightning coming off his roof. It was mid-January. My friend was removed by firemen from a steel radiator to which he appeared to have been welded. He's all right now, but on rainy days he claims to hear the audio portion of Channel 2 coming from a filling in a back tooth. Another friend blacked out four floors of her condominium building while attempting to connect a cable television line.

There must be a way to deal with this frustration. You might consider: going to a trade school to learn how to fix things yourself. In addition to solving your own problems, you will have a lucrative new career as one of the privileged few who know how to make things work and people wait. You will have more power than the chairman of AT&T.

CHAPTER NINE

It Calms the Nerves

The joke, like most, is told in various versions and has many fathers. I like the way Yiddish comedian Myron Cohen told it. He claimed to have overheard an older man say to his forty-years-younger companion at a Las Vegas nightclub, "Darling, if I lost all my money would you still love me?" "Of course I would," replied his Lolita, "and I'd miss you." Proving, in his case, that money *can* buy love. You simply had to hang on to it.

Perhaps I can help you hang on to what you have and add a little to it. My credentials: I started adult life as an economic illiterate, and thirty-five years later was written up in *Forbes* as an investment maven. I've squandered, wasted, and thrown away money, but I made it back and then some. Here are a few of the things I've learned.

Money is more important when you grow older. Not so much for what it will buy as for the demons it can banish. It is more potent than a twenty-year-old penis for men and acts as an aphrodisiac for the women they meet. Panic spells at four in the morning are quickly dissolved by contemplating thirty-year

Treasuries in the vault. The figures in the portfolio printout, if the market is up, can stir passions more deeply than the figures in *Penthouse*. You don't have to be rich to be financially secure. You do have to live artfully within your means. Many men with considerable means are strapped because they overspend. The worst afflication a man can have is a crazily extravagant wife. I'm grateful I fell in love with and married a somewhat stingy girl.

Women tend to spend more after they marry, but somewhat stingy women save more with the passing of each anxious year. How can you tell your prospective mate is stingy enough? I knew mine was when I discovered she'd bought a Mercedes-Benz for all cash on a secretary's salary. Anyway, that's what she told me.

What bliss to find such a mate. A girl I used to know (intimately) buried her bills so that a treasure hunt had to be organized to find them. I never knew what we owed until the sheriff arrived with an eviction notice and two of my cars were repossessed. It's hard to maintain an erection when your bed is collateral for a loan.

The stock market should be approached with more than the usual caution by the older man. If you do invest in stocks, do not—underscore *do not*—rely entirely on the advice of a broker. Perhaps they are called brokers because they can make you broker. While there are exceptions (my present broker, for example), I have found that their advice can be costly. They are, after all, judged to some extent by the amount of commissions whether you win or lose.

In any case, after fifty-five, start building up the income-producing portion of your portfolio. Put less emphasis on "growth" and more on dividends. Avoid "specs." Shift into high-grade municipal bonds when interest rates become attractive. Read the financial press carefully for news of excessive corporate salaries and perks. Proxy material, in particular, discloses what officers are taking from a company. A rule that's worked well for me is not to invest in companies where I'd be happy as an employee. They're probably giving away too much.

The best advice I ever read about stocks comes from the book *Where Are the Customers' Yachts?* by Fred Schwed, Jr. It was written nearly a half century ago. Advised Mr. Schwed:

When there is a stock-market boom, and everyone is scrambling for common stocks, take all your common stocks and sell them. Take the proceeds and buy conservative bonds. No doubt the stocks you sold will go higher. Pay no attention to this—just wait for the depression which will come sooner or later. When this depression—or panic—becomes a national catastrophe, sell out the bonds (perhaps at a loss) and buy back the stocks. No doubt the stocks will go still lower. Again pay no attention. Wait for the next boom. Continue to repeat this operation as long as you live, and you'll have the pleasure of dying rich.

For a newer and excellent guide to handling your money, I recommend John Train's *Preserving Capital*. It's capital!

In making any investment consider your age and probable life span. That lets out buying raw land for appreciation, building projects, or other budding businesses projected to come into profits well into the next century, anything with "long term" tacked on to its prospectus. As Lord Keynes said, "In the long term we're all dead." I never invest in anything that takes more than eighteen months or two years to make its move.

If you must buy a new house, never buy the best one in a poor neighborhood. The worst house in a rich neighborhood is always a superior investment. It's preferable to have your rich neighbors look down on you than your poor neighbors look up at you and throw rocks at your attack dogs. Probably you ought not to buy a house at all. Consider the income that you would receive from the money tied up in a house. You want mobility at your age. I decided not to buy a second home recently when I figured that the money required to buy it would, invested conservatively, bring in enough income for me to stay in any resort hotel I chose, with none of the headaches of home ownership and with my capital intact and liquid.

If you are, as I am, easily upset by complaints, it may not be a good idea for you to invest in rental property. A stock certificate or ninety-day Treasury bill does not call you up at three in the morning demanding a new toilet bowl. I have had to telephone plumbers from Nairobi to attend to demands of tenants on Long Island. The late, very rich and shrewd songwriter/producer Billy Rose advised, "Never buy anything that moves or needs paint."

Don't accept investment advice from doctors, and especially not from psychiatrists. My psychiatrist tried to interest me in investing in a submarine in the shape of a whale. The idea was that the whale of a submarine would surface off the beach at Santa Monica, California, and display advertising on its side. When I heard this idea I knew that transference had taken place. I was cured but he was ill. He did become rich later by "insanely" buying up every scrap of Malibu beachfront he could afford—proving another point. It doesn't hurt to be a little mad to make a lot of money.

Some personal investment advisers are far from infallible. In my experience their counsel is undistinguished at best. And, at worst, their advice can wipe you out. Work at managing your own money. Keep your own checkbook, even if it doesn't balance. Know where your money is going. Put it in businesses you understand, run if possible by people you know by reputation. If you have any rich friends, eavesdrop on their conversations. You may hear of some company move that will raise or depress a stock. Avoid stocks whose names begin with *Bio* or end in *ics* or *ix*. Before buying a stock always make certain the directors and officers or the company own more stock in it than you do. Wives of corporation directors who babble indiscreetly at lunch are a rich source of financial information. Listen carefully and buy them another drink.

Try not to lend money to friends. It's the best way, as Shakespeare wrote, to lose both money and friend. "If you would have enemies," states a Catalonian proverb, "lend money to your friends." And if you borrow, get it from a bank. A lender-friend will look disapprovingly at you each time you take a vacation or give a party.

I have different—and somewhat contradictory—rules for spending money.

Unless you're bone poor, always overtip. It makes life easier. Don't for a moment think it makes you appear gauche. No headwaiter, porter, or cabdriver ever shook his head while pocketing a twenty-dollar bill and said, "My God, he's gauche." *Au contraire.* Urban life is maddening and some restaurants are so crowded that it's life restoring to be able to get your favorite table at once. My wife swears that when I arrive at an airport, porters drop other people's baggage to pick up mine. I won't reveal how much I tip. That would be tacky. Just try increasing your gratuities until you get the desired results. It's not enough to tip generously. You must care about the people who serve you. Tips do not buy the right to be rude. Those who serve know more about good manners than most of those they serve. I'm treated well because I care for those who serve me. Tipping well is only one evidence of my concern for their welfare.

It's better to pick up the bill at dinner than outwait a friend who owes you one. Some people assume they are always your guests. If they think you are richer than they are, they're convinced they need never pay. There are elegant exceptions. A movie stuntman I know always brings flowers or a present when invited to my home and invariably wins the struggle to buy dinner when his turn comes up in a restaurant. Perhaps I'm prejudiced, but I find the more liberal politically someone is, the less likely he is to pick up a check. He may complain about big business but has no difficulty enjoying capitalist hospitality—yours.

A final word. Give presents but good ones. Here's another aphorism from Billy Rose: "If you only have five dollars to spend on a present, spend it on a bar of soap." Adjusted for inflation, that five dollars is now fifty dollars.

Don't spend everything you have because you don't want to outlive your money. Life is perverse. If you're broke, you'll live forever. If you're rich, you'll die tomorrow. To confound the fates, live it up, but little by little.

I think money—and living just below your means—are essential to staying young all your life. Having the shorts and living on the brink hasten the aging process, especially of your creditors. Money may not bring happiness, but it does calm the nerves.

CHAPTER TEN

Thanks for the Memory

You're panicked, humiliated, terrified. Standing next to you at a party is a woman. You can't remember her name. She's your wife. The next morning for one interminable minute you don't know where you are, who you are, and who the woman in your bed is.

These are the nightmare fears of the older man who's beginning to forget things. None of the above has actually occurred, but the older man worries that they will—to him.

To all of which I say, you're not beginning to forget things. You always did. You're simply beginning to notice it. All of us blank out on occasion and it's frightening. It's not the end of remembering.

When I was thirteen my mother would reprimand me by saying, "If your head were not on your body, you'd forget your head." I forgot my homework, failed to remember dental appointments, left my schoolbooks on the bus—in short, exhibited symptoms of senility prior to reaching puberty.

I mention this in defense of the idea that forgetfulness may be less an affliction of age than a defect of character. It is also, I believe, a symptom of brain overload. You've heard and remembered too much in your life, and some of it is relegated to the back burner of your mind. I am convinced we forget what (and whom) we want to forget. Who can ever forget the screen image of sunny, funny Marilyn Monroe? Other images are more easily discarded. When I was an officer candidate in World War II, I forgot where my company's barracks were and dismissed my men two miles away. It cost me my lieutenant bars. Young pilots have also had memory lapses and landed commercial planes at the wrong airports.

Training yourself to remember names—at any age—is difficult. Some people don't make it easier. The worst are those who leave you hanging with "You don't remember me, do you?" I'm tempted to reply, "No, I don't, but what have you done to make me forget you?"

Unless you're a world-class celebrity, it is always considerate to open a conversation with "I'm so-and-so." Invariably the person so addressed will respond with his or her name. I've found that even celebrities will sometimes take you off the hook. Mary Tyler Moore, one of the more visible people in the world, says, "I'm Mary Tyler Moore." Johnny Carson and Tony Randall (among others) are not above identifying themselves.

One of the most engaging examples of this trait occurred years ago in an elevator at New York's Radio City Music Hall. Extending his hand to the page who was escorting him to his seat, the other occupant of the car said, "Hello. I'm Dwight D. Eisenhower."

But what if you haven't (and aren't given) a clue as to the identity of the man who is pumping your hand amiably? I usually finesse the situation by asking, "What are you up to these days?" This may trigger the memory, but there are dangers. The reply may be "I'm John McEnroe and I've just returned from Wimbledon." If someone thinks *you* are somebody else— or obviously is mistaken in saying he saw you someplace or talked to you—don't correct him.

I've tried memorizing faces, especially when I've committed a social gaffe. I failed repeatedly to recognize one famous lady who invariably recognized me. In frustration she exclaimed, "Why, you don't know who I am, do you, David?" I took a shot in the dark, blurting out the name of a lookalike who was twenty years younger. Flattered by being mistaken for a young woman, she forgave me. I determined I would never again forget her. A few weeks later, in a Manhattan restaurant, a friend waved me over to introduce me to a woman who'd been sitting directly in my line of sight for the previous two hours. I hadn't had a clue that it was the lady I'd vowed never to forget.

As a consequence I am mildly anxious whenever I patronize a restaurant whose clients are well known to everyone but me. It is no fun fumbling for the name Tom Cruise when everyone around you is oohing and aahing at the handsome young man who has stopped to talk to you. Elaine's and the Russian Tea Room, Manhattan's premier celebrity stops, are filled with land mines for the forgetful of the famous, and I rarely venture there without my wife, who still remembers the name of the second assistant director on *Ben Hur*. Or was it *Ben Him*?

It is possible to overcome some memory problems by adopting a few stratagems.

Try running down the alphabet to see if a letter triggers a last name. If you get the last name, chances are you'll remember the first. Sometimes running down the letters may provide sudden memory vibes. Keep repeating them in your mind until your memory is finally jogged. *Voilà*, the name!

When in a restaurant or club, try to avoid gazing at someone who looks familiar but whose name does not immediately come to mind. If she waves a kiss at you, ask the headwaiter to give you her name. He probably knows her and you'll be able to greet her properly. If a man waves, the reservation is probably in his name—easy to find out.

At sit-down dinner parties go to your assigned table and look carefully at the place cards—particularly to the right and left of you. Glance at the chart or list indicating guests at other tables. You'll be able to match the names to the faces if the list is not too big, or if you don't forget the names on your way to your table.

At cocktail parties join a group engaged in conversation. Sooner or later someone will refer to "old Charlie, here," or, better still, a round of introductions will be made that you will overhear.

On an airplane, check with the flight attendant for the name of the attractive woman across the aisle who appears to know you.

As for appointments and social engagements, keep double lists. Write your appointments in your diary and make certain your secretary's diary and your wife's social calendar conform. It is very embarrassing to forget a social engagement or to get the wrong date. On one occasion years ago (age was not the factor), my wife and I arrived at a dinner pary one week early. Our future hosts were not amused.

Perhaps the most irritating and persistent problem of forgetfulness has to do with things, not people. Keys, umbrellas, combs, and other small items are constantly being lost. My wife has a habit of taking off her earrings and forgetting where she put them. We have crawled under tables of Paris bistros and under seats of Land-Rovers in Botswana in vain efforts to find these trinkets.

As for failing to remember what people have said to you, perhaps in a business meeting, there is no substitute for keeping a notepad of reminders. My difficulty is remembering where I put the notepad. Lately I have asked my secretary of thirty years to keep my list of reminders herself, but she forgets to remind me of them. I thought I had solved the problem by getting her a blackboard, but she never looks at it. Meanwhile, I have accumulated dozens of thick little pocket notebooks, complete with Cartier pencils, while I continue to make notes on the back of envelopes. Which I lose— *both* the notebooks with Cartier pencils *and* the backs of envelopes. I have also enlisted computers—the pocket size—to jog my memory. Too cumbersome. My programming is fallible.

What I hate most about forgetting is the lack of control it suggests. Lost objects take on a significance far greater than their value. The maddening thing is that a few days or weeks later I recall exactly where I misplaced the beloved object. My wife can almost see the precious brooch she dropped on the floor of a San Francisco taxi while getting out. I can remember where I put my grandfather's cuff links in a Buenos Aires hotel room, but I cannot recall how or why I left them there.

When you have lost something of value, it is best to retrace your steps. Sometimes that is exceedingly difficult. My wife hid some jewelry in a pair of old shoes, forgot she had done so, and tossed the old shoes into the trash. At four o'clock one morning she and a kindly apartment-house employee went through mountains of trash and—*voilà*! found the gems sparkling amid the garbage.

I discovered I had misplaced my passport while en route to the airport in Paris. I returned to the George V hotel, secured entrance to movie mogul Darryl F. Zanuck's suite, where I had had a meeting, crawled under chairs and tables, and found nothing. A friend suggested I forget discretion and confess that my passport might be in some flat where I spent the night with—let's not worry about it—some woman. Call her, he urged. Alas, I had dined alone that evening on the Left Bank, and telephoned the restaurant—nothing. As I was aimlessly wandering around the George V lobby, a light went on in my head. I remembered having been in a drugstore on the

Champs Élysées. As soon as I entered, the saleswoman exclaimed, *"Voilà votre passport."* I had left it on the counter while buying perfume for my wife.

Today I no longer turn the house upside down to retrieve a comb. I buy another. I purchase many umbrellas and pens—so I can lose some. I still keep a checklist of what I am carrying—keys, wallet, money clip—and periodically pat my pocket to see if they are there. Sometimes they are not. I go crazy.

Short-term memory fades with advancing years, but memory for the past improves. The human computer is inundated by the trivia of decades, but those early memories—of that girl, the first job, or college graduation—are clear. Smells are a potent memory stirrer. Hot tar will instantly summon up vivid images of my youth on Long Island when roads melted under the summer sun. A whiff of Arpège, and a woman I loved forty years ago materializes, her gown, coiffure, and smile as they were at twenty.

Who cares if you can't remember what you had for dinner last night? Perhaps it wasn't memorable. I'll wager you can remember a dozen that were. Insanity was once defined as remembering everything at once. Thanks for the memory—singular.

There's something else I meant to put in this chapter, but for the life of me I can't remember what it was.

CHAPTER ELEVEN

The Only Cure for Depression

When I mentioned to my wife that I was going to write about not being depressed as you get older, she first looked funny, then tried to sweep funny off her face, then composed herself, then lost the battle and said, "*You*? A book about not being depressed as you get older? That's like Richard Nixon writing the definitive history of the Harlem Dance Theater or Madonna redefining Bach. . . . I have seen you *terminally* depressed as recently as yesterday." "Yes," I said, "but didn't you see me *unterminally* depressed a few hours later? It never lasts, does it? I come out okay every time, don't I?"

That's the point. You will come out okay every time. How to endure the pain is the sermon for today. No book, including this one, can tell you how to get undepressed. Oh, we've all heard that exercise will do it—if it doesn't give you cardiac arrest. Eating, some claim, is an antidepressant, but getting fat isn't. Others advise us to get out of the house and be with people. How depressing. That only results in the greater strain of having to act happy when you're not. I do have suggestions that may work, however, so don't leave me.

Winston Churchill referred to depression as the Black Dog and suggested you get out of the way of family and friends until *it* slinks away. And slink away it will—or it can kill you. The latter is extremely unlikely, however, unless you are terminally ill (a good reason to be depressed).

Everyone, even including giddy Goldie Hawn, gets depressed. You may blame your own depression on growing older, but you will be wrong. Teenage suicide is rampant. Many years ago, a song titled "Gloomy Sunday" caused young lovers to kill themselves. You may even blame your depression on not having enough money, unless you reflect on the sad, alienated, drug-ridden lives of so many of the rich and temporarily famous.

Depression spares no class, age, or gender. Its cure, short of drug treatment, has proven as elusive as the cure for the common cold. I can try, however, to show you my way to treat its symptoms.

I think I was always depressed until recently. I was almost suicidal in my teens because I knew my beloved grandfather would soon die, and later during the breakup of two marriages, and hundreds of times in between, including all Christmases and New Year's Eves. I grew up in the Depression, which, during those formative years, may have given me the idea.

I'm aware that some of my depressed episodes were situational—that is, something real was getting me down. However, I'm convinced that something real doesn't always get you down. I don't recall a single bout of depression during my four years in the army, even when I was scrubbing latrines and sleeping in frozen foxholes. I rarely reflected on the irony of my situation. In a single day I had gone from the privileged life of editor of a national magazine to the lower-depths existence of an army private. I had no time to brood about my drastically lowered status or the possibility of sudden death. I'm told combat marines in action also do not experience depression. They are too busy staying alive.

Too busy staying alive. That's the key. And that's what I think older people ought to be doing. Depression has little to do with a root cause. It took me more than sixty years to find that out. I had experienced depression during what should have been my happiest times. The better the news, the worse I would feel. And after fours years of psychoanalysis I was often more depressed than ever.

All this illustrates that depression can strike whether the news is good or bad . . . and, as one who has kept Churchill's Black Dog as a household pet, I've concluded that constant, even frenetic activity is the best way to keep that howling dog away.

That means you must be too busy: reading, writing (as I am now), walking, working, arguing, gardening, helping (other victims of depression), loving, suing, eating (sometimes the best preventive), but definitely *not* drinking, smoking, or drugging.

Sometimes depression will break through despite

your busyness. When it does, *let* yourself be depressed. Clear out the house. Cover the furniture. Send your wife or lover to the movies and your grandchildren to camp. Put the cat and dogs in a kennel. Then sit alone in your room thinking the darkest, dreariest, most forlorn thoughts. Get it out. Cry. Scream. Break a few dishes (careful with the good china). Soon, sooner than you think, you will get so bloody bored with your dark thoughts that you will pull the blinds up, open the window (with nary a thought of jumping out), and breathe deeply.

The miracle is that no matter how bad things continue to be, the healthy human mind is incapable of sustaining negative thoughts for an indefinite period.

CHAPTER TWELVE

When You Need Your Head Examined

"Anyone who sees a psychiatrist ought to have his head examined," proclaimed the late Sam Goldwyn. The trouble is, very few candidates for psychiatry do have their heads examined. Had that extraordinary composer George Gershwin done so, his brain tumor might have been discovered and removed and with it the symptoms that led to the couch.

However, there are times when all the other root causes can be ruled out and the psychiatrist, the referral of last resort for many doctors, offers the best and only hope for relief of emotional agony. What drove me into psychoanalysis the first time was the pain of a failed marriage.

I had always hated the idea of psychiatry. I mocked it. I thought it was for the weak and self-obsessed. I was right—because nobody was weaker and more self-obsessed than I. After the shock of having been abandoned by my second wife had immobilized me, I sought psychiatry as a painkiller, as a drug. I remember lying in despair on a couch in my office

—it *was* a point of honor never to miss a day's work—when my friend Ernest Lehman came in and observed my distress. See somebody, he said. And I did.

I found my psychoanalyst in the Yellow Pages. I went down the list of medical specialists until I found my man—Mark L. Stone, M.D., a diplomate of the American Board of Psychiatry and, best of all, on Beverly Drive in Beverly Hills, a ten-minute drive from my office at the Twentieth Century Fox studios.

Dr. Stone, a moon-faced man who had served his internship in mental hospitals, was becoming bored with the hang-ups of the rich and famous. He eventually quit his practice and became a successful real estate investor. He prospered, but it was a loss for his patients. He was a skilled and sensitive physician. I was his challenge for a time—an expensive one, as property values were going up and he deferred going into real estate while treating me. He even cosigned my loan agreements to keep me in treatment.

My experience was both unique and typical. It was unique because there was a finishing point for me; unlike many, I could free myself from my therapist. (I've often thought dependency to be part of the illness.) And it was typical in that not everything is curable. The more stubborn problem—in my case, fear of doctors—remains unresolved.

Psychoanalysis is not for all. It is not for the financially strapped. Today's fees of a hundred and fifty dollars for a forty-five-minute hour in many cities adds to the patient's already severe anxiety. It is ineffective in dealing with alcoholism and it can't get you a job, although it may help you discover why you can't find one. Don't rely upon it to find someone to love unless it is yourself you want to love, always the first step.

Psychiatry is effective in guiding you in your relationships with others. It reduces anxiety and helps you to identify irrational fears. Dealing with irrational fears constructively is something else. It's not easy—and often not possible. The psychiatrist, if you have been lucky in your choice, can be your friend, the one to whom you confide what you can't tell anyone else. True, you have to pay for this trust, but I have found there is always a measure of unpurchasable love and friendship in a good doctor-patient relationship. The priest will impose moral or religious strictures in exchange for absolution; your wife may consider your malaise a form of criticism of her. Only the psychiatrist will not judge you.

It is natural to think of the psychiatrist as a friend who will continue to love you after treatment is over. Why not extend a paid friendship into an unpaid one? Here's why not. Psychiatrists are an odd lot, really, and I say that with affection. To spend all day having people dump on you can warp the off-duty personality. As a group I have found them rather like members of the clergy. They want to have a good time, but what will others think? I once wandered into a group of psychiatrists on vacation. They were extremely stiff, something like the British at play as observed by the French.

These arbiters of innermost fears seem more comfortable among their own. Part of their unease may be due to their need to remain authority figures. I think it's best to break off the relationship when you leave treatment, and most psychiatrists do so for their sake as well as for the good of their patients.

As to whether you need a psychiatrist at all, the rule I have applied to myself is to go when the pain of not going is too great. If you are able to work out your problems on your own, even with some pain, that is probably the best and most lasting therapy. But don't be a hero. Everyone has a breaking point, and some problems are beyond your ability to cope.

Quite apart from helping you deal with emotional problems, there's something to be said for psychiatry as a learning experience. I was told to look upon psychoanalysis as an investment of time and money comparable to a college education. And so it was. You, too, may have studied everything but yourself, and you needn't go into analysis to complete the course. There are newer, more pragmatic, and less expensive forms of therapy available today.

The benefits of treatment can continue throughout life. Finally, there is something even better than a voyage into yourself and that is a voyage out of yourself. Neurotics are preoccupied with self, permanent members of the "me" generation. If you can interest yourself in others, your problems may disappear. The later years are the best times to give more than one takes from life. They are the teaching years, the mentor years. "Adopt" someone who needs your guidance and wisdom. Helping somebody other than yourself is the best way I've found to deflect the dragons of the gathering night.

CHAPTER THIRTEEN

Should Auld Acquaintance Be Forgot? Sometimes, Yes

I believe it was Ambrose Bierce, a cynic's cynic, who said, "A friend in need is no friend." I know it was Bierce who, in his infamous *Devil's Dictionary*, defined happiness as "an agreeable sensation arising from contemplating the misery of another." And in Hollywood, where friendship is as enduring as an ice cube in a sauna, the words go like this: "It is not enough that your friend not succeed; he must also fail."

Behind these dismal aphorisms lies a scintilla of truth. We are not always our best friend's best friend. We *are* too often jealous and hoping secretly that things do not turn out too well for him. It's more exciting when disaster is in the air, and it's *his* disaster. Fortunately, these dark yearnings remain hidden, or friendship would be as rare as Brontosaurus.

Notwithstanding one's secret thoughts, friends must be valued. Like plants, they require care. They can become true friends if one understands the realities and dynamisms of the relationship.

Old friends are often the best, but not always. You can't rewrite history with an old friend. He knows you. If you've been saying you fought in the Tet offensive, you have to worry that this "friend" will reveal that the only battle you took part in was in Manhattan . . . in a bar. He may also disclose that you didn't go to Yale and are Ukrainian instead of being descended from Thomas Jefferson. But the truth that an old friend knows is your continuity with the long ago. Possibly he has known you longer than your wife (or wives) and children. He may even have known your parents. It is reassuring that he is here, whatever the present terms of your friendship. I have one friend I have known since childhood and he is like no other friend. We have memories to keep alive our departed friends and families. It is almost a holy bond.

Sadly, old friends can become obsolete in this harried world. Long friendships are like some long marriages. The ties that bound you may have long since unraveled. This is particularly true of college classmates whom college brought together and graduation flung apart. Even longtime business associates may fade away when they leave jobs. The work is the mortar that holds many such friendships together. When that is gone, friends become acquaintances.

There are other perils to long friendships. Sudden success of one friend can cause stress. As Wilfrid Sheed put it in an essay, you must "make a real effort to appear to rejoice when a friend succeeds." Finally, true feelings surface, usually months later. "You've changed," laments the less fortunate one. "No," responds the luckier one, "*You've* changed—in your attitude toward me." Often all too true and too bad.

You may not always be the "lucky one." Whether your life has been a romp to success or, as is more likely, an up-and-down affair with more disappointment than triumphs, your friends will be fewer as you grow older. Death takes some. Changes in your work environment remove others with whom your only common interest was the job. This shrinkage is especially traumatic when you "retire" from a company. You, then, may well become the "dropped one."

You *will* need friends after your acquisitive years. Loneliness is a killer. Some old friends may have been discarded by you, or you may have been abandoned by them. The remedy is clear. Make new friends who accept you as you now are and hang on to those old friends you still have who knew you as you were.

I've recommended that you let a woman into your life, preferably more than one. Now is a good time to make women friends. They will welcome a man in their lives—there being so few of you. A recent study finds that having a confidante actually reduces depression, so common in the older, adrift male.

One reason I've also advocated that you work yourself to death is that your new friends, whether men or women—like your old—are most likely to be found in your workplace. You have to court them. As Emerson pointed out, "The only way to have a friend is to be one." If your work is not in an office but in your home or a studio, get to know your suppliers or your lawyer or accountant. A world-class writer who lives in an isolated New England village has found his postman to be more interesting and learned than some of his literary chums in New York. Everyone suffers loneliness, and a dinner invitation will be eagerly received.

Seek young friends. I've found younger men enjoy the benefits of knowing older people. Besides, it will help keep you young. John Kluge, the immensely successful entrepreneur, now in his seventies, credits some of his incredible drive and energy to his association with those younger than he.

Make a friend of your wife, if you have one. It's astonishing how many men ignore their most proximate and available source of comradeship. She may be aching to be treated as a friend instead of as a wife. Show her the courtesy and consideration you would a new friend and she will become a new friend, maybe even a new lover.

There is an art to keeping friends as well as making friends. Do not mistake friendship as a license to tell the truth. More pain has been inflicted by indiscriminate truth-telling than by lies. Honesty too often means being hurtful and wounding someone. As long as you keep true counsel with yourself, it doesn't hurt if you dissemble with a friend. White lies are told a lot in heaven. "Unvarnished truth" is going around a lot in hell. The test is, would telling the truth help? As Wilfrid Sheed wrote, "I can dispense right away with the friend who tells you things for your own good." Usually, all it does is lose a friend.

False friends have their uses too. I take no offense

when a "friend" drops away because he finds I can no longer help him. When I ceased to be a powerful mogul in Hollywood, an important agent I considered a friend did not call me until I was restored to power years later. At least our relationship was clear. I had no illusions about it. He was a true "false" friend. We resumed our false friendship without recrimination on my part or explanation on his.

Be a clown, but if you can't be one, become friends with someone who makes you laugh or fascinates you with his stories. Such men or women are always seeking an audience. Bernard Berenson once said, "A friend is someone who stimulates me and to whom I am stimulated to talk. When the stimulation no longer occurs, it is a spent and exhausted friendship and continues as a burden and a bore."

I don't agree with Berenson that every friend need be a spellbinder. There's something good to be said for mild bores—not the terminal kind who have you gasping for relief but the kind who make few demands on your attention. Such bores may even act as a soporific and lull you to sleep. A semibore promotes tranquility and saves you the energy of being "on." You needn't be at your peak. It's comforting to have a friend who requires little effort on your part except to be there. At times in one's life sitting in comparative silence with such a companion can be extraordinarily restful and recuperative.

There are also friends who perform a service—perhaps he's business-oriented and you're a culture maven, in which case he advises you on investments and you tell him which plays to see. There are also those friends so removed from your world that you can confide in them without fear of betrayal. You may even get an objective view of a family or business problem that you could not get from someone closer to the scene.

I've always kept separate sets of friends who do not know each other. I did this even in my youth. The friends who saw me off to college were jealous of one another because most of them hadn't known another set of friends existed.

Today, still, many of my friends do not know one another. They live in separate worlds, but my world encompasses them all.

You can reestablish an old friendship after years of separation. The circumstances that thrust you apart—marriage, young children, career demands, and so on—may no longer exist and you can resume the relationship. These old friends are a living link to a "previous life" when you were both young.

There is a purity in true friendships, whether new or old. We mourn their passing with special grief.

Some of my best friends are dead. They never grow older. I think of them as I fall asleep and relive our times together. There's Charles, my best friend at Stanford, who wrote shortly after graduation, "I want everything to stay as it is so that nothing will change." Nothing did change for Charles. He died soon afterward. And Elliot, from whom I was inseparable in high school, never reached twenty, killed in a training accident in World War II. It is interesting to imagine what his life would have been like if he had lived. Instead, he was destined to be untouched by the aches, creaks, and anxieties of advancing age. I have known girls too—gone before their prime, never to be thickened or lined but still slim and beautiful as they made their exit. In a somber moment I think they have been spared the worst of times, but then my adrenaline flows and I still believe the best is yet to be—and would have been for them.

By keeping fresh the memory of long departed friends, you can recreate your own youthful buoyancy and optimism, the conviction that anything is possible. These are friends who will never disappoint you and are never truly lost. They are still missed. Nothing more poignantly expresses the spirit of youthful friendship than these lines by the Greek poet Callimachus:

> *They told me, Heraclitus,*
> *They told me you were dead;*
> *They brought me bitter news to hear*
> *And bitter tears to shed.*
> *I wept as I remembered*
> *How often you and I*
> *Had tired the sun with talking*
> *And sent it down the sky.*

You will indeed be lucky to have had such a friendship, but whether "false" or true, all friendships are essential to a vibrant later life. Cultivate them, whatever their label, and watch both of you grow.

CHAPTER FOURTEEN

Etiquette for the Older Man

Some (but not all) of my rules of etiquette apply as much to the young as to the old. They are a personal guide to social behavior and not intended to be "the law."

The suggestions are hardly all-inclusive, but perhaps set the tone for behavior in situations not included. The tone is be your best self.

I am indebted to George Axelrod, playwright, for this advice: If you must break off a love affair, do so in a good restaurant where any woman with a shred of social ambition would not think of making a scene.

Always be on the telephone before someone you have called is on the line.

Do not ask your secretary to make your social engagements. She may get the dates wrong. Written invitations followed by written reminders are de rigueur.

Address others by their first names after a modicum of social exchange. It is stuffy to do otherwise. Don't protest when someone half your age continues to address you formally. Accept it gracefully as a sign of respect.

A gentleman extends the same courtesy to all, regardless of station. George Bernard Shaw expressed this brilliantly in these remarks in *Pygmalion*: "The great secret is not having bad manners or good manners or any other particular sort of manners, but having the same manners for all human souls. The question is not whether I treat you rudely, but whether you ever heard me treat anyone else better."

When you fail to show up for a luncheon or dinner party because of forgetfulness or a mistaken diary entry, send flowers and a note of explanation and apology. Then put it behind you. Continued remorseful protestations will make matters worse—and boring.

Never be the first to arrive at a party or the last to go home and never, never be both.

Always dance with the least prepossessing lady at your table. When you are dancing with someone younger and stronger, be abandoned in short bursts, then slow down as a gentleman of your age of necessity must do. Don't get carried away or you may be carried away.

Keep dinner table conversation brief. Anything more than a few minutes of banter may cause your dinner companion's eyes to glaze over. By that time you may be required to whip your head around to your other companion because *her* eyes are glazing over.

Be careful not to impart your wisdom to a guest whose background you do not know. You may be instructing a Nobel laureate in his own field.

Some social gaffes are inevitable. When violent

arguments develop among guests, usually one of them leaves and sends flowers. Most gaffes are forgiven but never forgotten. Still, they do bring a dull party to life.

Always send notes, flowers, or an unusual foxy gift after a small dinner party. Hostesses never tire of being told how grand it was. The gift must be carefully selected—exactly the right Bordeaux for an oenophile, a rare book for a bibliophile.

As a guest you are also under some obligation to return hospitality with a party of your own.

When you have been fired, divorced, or the object of scandalous publicity, consider Arnold Bennett's advice: "Always behave as if nothing has happened." That is the time to act so that others will be in a tizzy because you are not falling apart.

Send a lady with whom you have spent the night flowers and a note—especially if the romance is doomed. Always leave before breakfast unless you are in love, so that the subject of commitment need not be raised.

A woman willing to be kissed on the lips lets it be known by leaning slightly forward. I have never been mistaken about this.

Give generous gratuities to the cook and servants when you are a houseguest. Do so well before you leave so that your hosts will not notice. Forty or fifty dollars for the cook and twenty for the maid is in order for a long weekend.

Money talks—and therefore *you* need not speak of it. Even the Fool in Shakespeare's *King Lear* counseled, "Have more than thou showest."

In declining a social engagement it is best to tell the truth. It is acceptable to say you are tired or have three other dates that week and can't handle a fourth. It is cruel and unforgivable to cancel an engagement because a "better" one has come along. "Trade up" only if invited to a state dinner at the White House. Never ask for a list of the other guests. If you are sufficiently important or interesting, a hostess will supply one.

Do not be vague if you are serious about inviting someone. Do not say, "Let's see how we all feel about having dinner Sunday." This leaves one not knowing what to do about Sunday. Say, "Eight P.M. at Mortimer's. We'll meet there."

It's fine to invite someone to lunch on the same day but unpardonable to cancel on the same day.

Gossiping is delicious, but beware of repeating anything that may destroy a marriage or a career, unless that is your goal. Be especially wary of passing along rumors about prominent persons. Irv Kupcinet, the Chicago columnist, aptly remarked on a Phil Donahue television show, "The sexual perferences of certain celebrities should remain a secret among the three of them." Besides, gossip has a way of revealing its source, and you may lose a friend or gain a lawsuit.

Even a reasonably interesting person owes it to his host to "bone up" and sing for his supper; one of the perils of small gatherings is that you must try to give good guest.

Always go to the bathroom before sitting down to dinner. It will spare your getting up.

I have yet to find the woman, however liberated,

who does not revel in having a door opened, a seat offered, or an arm extended to help her across the street. Women, especially now, like to be treated with deference because there are so few men who do so—and, perhaps, because there are so few men.

Women who use foul language are embarrassing, especially if there are gentlemen present.

The new etiquette decrees that you refrain from smoking in public, but women are more likely to be offenders than men. Let them. If you also have the habit, be grateful for a wife who shares your addiction or at least tolerates it. I went through two marriages before I found a woman who liked my cigars and the result has been a long, happy, and smoke-filled marriage.

Amy Vanderbilt correctly stated that breakfast is the one meal at which it is perfectly good manners to read the newspaper.

When you spill something, let someone else clean up the mess. Treat the incident with the same élan as you did while a sloppy teenager.

Show your family the courtesy you would a stranger, no matter how trying that may be. The Chinese hold that in a good marriage a husband and wife regard each other as guests.

If you have hearing problems and are too vain to wear a hearing aid, don't ask "What?" more than once. If you fail to hear something a second time, fake it and change the subject.

As for turning down requests for money, time, and other scarce commodities, do so decisively. T. S. Eliot observed, "The years between fifty and seventy are the hardest . . . You are always being asked to do things, and yet you are not decrepit enough to turn them down . . ." Turn them down.

Be brisk with your good-byes, unhurried with your hellos, sparse with flattery, and profuse with expressions of love.

When someone is unpardonably rude, take no notice and go on as if nothing had occurred. Slowly remove yourself, so slowly that the offender will not know you are gone and will continue sputtering to someone else.

In general, Epicetus's advice holds as well now as it did in ancient times: "Compare thyself in life as at a banquet. If a plate is offered thee, extend thy hand and take it moderately; if it is to be withdrawn, do not detain it. If it comes to thy side, make not thy desire loudly known, but wait patiently until it be offered thee."

To which I would add, always say thank you. It is the essence of good manners in all but the bleakest circumstances.

CHAPTER FIFTEEN

Getting Away

After fifty, one of the few things people do more of is travel. All it takes is a passport, a visa, and a credit card to book space on the Orient or Trans-Siberian express. Romantically inclined travelers should be warned, however, that they are less likely to encounter sinister-looking men in trench coats than little old ladies with walkers.

Why travel, especially when you are older and tireder? Simple. You have more time and, usually, more money. You're also more likely to be bored.

Even if you're still working, travel on your own can be a means of shaking off disappointment, grief, or depression. Your troubles may be patiently waiting for you when you return, but you'll have fresh energy with which to confront them. Noel Coward put it elegantly in "Sail Away": "When the wind and the weather blow your dreams sky high,/Sail away, sail away." A first-class seat at thirty-seven thousand feet can sometimes be better than a psychiatrist's couch for sorting out priorities, especially if there is a drink and a bowl of nuts within reach. Sometimes there's also a scare along the way to jar you into realizing

what's important. On my world trip I was awakened
by a sickening downdraft that almost plunged our
aircraft into the shark-filled Indian Ocean. For five
interminable minutes we rocked and careened while
lightning put flame on our wings. We experienced
most of the sensations of going down in a plane
crash. My career problems then became unimportant—and they still are.

Even uneventful travel puts problems in perspective. From the moment the aircraft pushes back from
the gate, you are in another habitat, temporarily sev-
ered from earthly concerns. To those on the ground
you're but flashing lights moving across the sky.

For nomads who are dehumanized by strapped-in
air travel, battered by delays at the baggage carousel, a
sea voyage is a tonic, offering a peaceful and beautiful
place to reassess one's life situation and the opportunity to lose oneself in the company of strangers.
Though costly in time and money, it is body-, soul-,
and mind-restoring.

The sea is also an aphrodisiac, although you will
have to work harder to attract a good-looking woman
aboard ships because there will be more competition
than on land. There is, however, a great opportunity
for a brief but beautiful encounter.

If you are one of those who agree with Samuel
Johnson that "being in a ship is being in a jail, with
the chance of being drowned," then perhaps travel by
train is your only alternative. Except for the Orient
Express and South Africa's Blue train, however, trains

today, even Japan's Bullet and France's TGV super-expresses, are no longer particularly luxurious. Meals are served airline style at your seat and it's too rocky to walk around.

Another form of travel, becoming increasingly appealing each year, is to head to one place—the Tuscany region of Italy, for example—by the most comfortable means and *stay* there for the duration of your holiday, straying only to nearby attractions.

Just a few suggestions for travel anywhere:

My scheme for packing is simple. Imagine your naked body, if the thought is not too depressing. Then start dressing it from the ground up, so to speak. First, socks and shoes—how many pairs will you need? Usually three, including what you will be wearing. One for dress, two for walking, plus slippers. Undershorts, undershirts, pants, shirts, sweaters, ties, cuff links follow. Outer garments come next. A raincoat will double for a topcoat. Once you have your basic wardrobe checklist completed, you can move on to toilet articles, reading matter, money, passport (visas in order?), tickets. These latter items should be left on top of your packed baggage. (Pack not later than the night before.) Forget the advice about traveling light. It's better to check your major baggage than to get a hernia carrying it. You may end up traveling lighter later when one or more pieces are lost. Not to worry. I have never lost anything permanently in a lifetime of travel. It always turns up in forty-eight hours or less. What doesn't turn up are items stolen out of unlocked zipper compartments. Designer luggage is more likely to be pilfered than the cheaper, unbranded variety. Beware of pickpockets in every airport and keep hand baggage in your hands or pressed between your feet when you stop at a ticket counter.

If you are an anxious traveler, you might consider a separate small bag containing those hard-to-be-without items you will need in the event that your baggage is delayed in reaching you. This might include a couple of shirts and pairs of underwear, toilet articles, medicine, and a couple of pairs of socks.

As for the journey, observe Samuel Johnson's advice:

> Turn all care out of your head as soon as
>   you mount the chaise.
> Do not think about frugality;
>   your health is worth more than it can cost.
> Do not continue any day's journey to fatigue.
> Take now and then a day's rest.
> Cast away all anxiety; and keep your mind easy.

That means you needn't worry whether you've turned the gas off. It will be burning when you return, and like Phileas Fogg's errant manservant, Passepartout, you will pay. But for now, play Nero. Let it burn while you fiddle.

When your return flight is canceled, you are, under certain circumstances, entitled to free transportation on the next available flight. If you are delayed overnight, your hotel and food expenses will be paid. Once, during a holiday in Britain, my Air India flight to New York was three days late. Air India cheerfully refunded the cost of an extra three days at London's elegant Claridge's plus a small New Year's Eve party. That's class—or rather first class—on Air India.

Take soap to most destinations. Soap bars are miniscule in some of the best hotels of Europe.

Sweaters are necessary on an airplane. Cabin temperature can fall quite rapidly even in tropic zones. Outside your cabin window it's fifty degrees below zero.

Buy the foreign currency you need at a major New York, San Francisco, Chicago, or Los Angeles bank. You'll get a better rate and not have to fumble with exchanging your money on arrival for tips and taxis.

Take a Bible. You might get to know and like this remarkable book during a long flight. You might even need to use it.

If you're traveling with your spouse, avoid arguments on the way to the airport. For some reason relationships become fragile when you're about to take a trip.

Do not put personal belongings or documents in the pocket in front of your seat. They tend to remain there when you deplane. You are most likely to lose things after a long flight when you are zonked out.

Bring toilet paper. At your age you never know when you'll need it or where. I was caught in Egypt without the proverbial pot. Panic led me to consider an open tomb, but a desert facility turned out not to be a mirage and had plumbing that did not date from Ramses II.

Do not drink the local water anywhere but home. If bottled water is not available, drink the local beer. As for India, tropical islands, and other places where the food can be of dubious origin, stick to cooked meals and fruit that can be peeled (bananas, pineapple, et cetera), but wash your hands after discarding the peel. Avoid ice cream, cheese, and other dairy products.

Third world countries are recommended only to those with an unflappable disposition, a cast-iron stomach, and a sadomasochistic bent. Go once, anyway, for the adventure and the hell of it.

Italy is especially hospitable to Americans, and you can live happily there forever, particularly with an Italian woman. Beware, however, of her tendency to gain weight. Pasta has destroyed more than one fine romance. Germany can be a surprise, particularly Hamburg, that Hanseatic city with some of the most beautiful women in Europe and the best food. German women are hearty and they adore older men. Munich is fine, too, but Berlin is still grave and gray, lacking the abandon of the years of which Christopher Isherwood wrote in his *Berlin Stories*.

What can you say about Paris that Cole Porter has not already said? Porter loved Paris even when it drizzled and sizzled. It is an impossible, vain, and blasé city, like a woman who has been adored too long. Paris is voyeuristic. Everybody watches. If I were alone at my age, I would live in Paris, where men are never too old for love. I would bring money. The

Frenchwomen I have known can scent a man with money as readily as their dogs can sniff out a pound of red meat. They are chic and funny and wonderful, well worth an old man's gold.

London is particularly suited for those who miss the civility and formality of the past. The class system is alive and well. As for British women, they are no longer plain wrens. Like London's food, British women have improved measurably in the postwar years, and the children and grandchildren of the Blitz are alluring and stylish. Best of all, unlike their Paris counterparts, they can be wildly romantic because they are still a bit naive. They are not so earthy-sexy as the Germans and Scandinavians, but they are talented.

Given all this information, you may still decide not to venture abroad. But before you decide there's no place like home, I urge you to look elsewhere. At the least you may find yourself.

CHAPTER SIXTEEN

Potpourri

Many of us become pains in the ass as we grow older.

Years ago, my wife and I visted Jean Paul Getty at his Sutton Place estate outside London. We were there because the world's richest man wanted advice about women from my wife. "Why," he asked, "do I have so much difficulty establishing a harmonious relationship with a woman?" My wife responded with another question. "Why, Mr. Getty, do you insist on associating with women one-third your age?" Mr. Getty replied slowly, "Because, Mrs. Brown, older women are too difficult."

So are older men.

Some of them tend to go on about how much better everything used to be. Boring.

Many older people ramble interminably until their trapped listeners are ready to kill. Be brief and brisk (but never brusque).

Repeating the same stories does not improve them. Keep track of their use and retire them after a few weeks.

You're often angry. You don't know at what. It

surfaces in bursts of ill temper. Try to curb becoming combative, argumentative, or overopinionated.

Rigidity is a particularly unattractive sign of growing old. Save it for rigor mortis. Learn to say, "Why not?" instead of "Why?"

Wear today's styles. Leave slobbery to the young while you adopt the new snobbery. Be fastidious but not trendy.

Don't take forever to get yourself to go out. You'll be astonished to learn how much faster you can move if you try—and it's good exercise.

Unfinished Business

To make yourself more resilient, reflect on the things you haven't done—the unfinished business of your life. Here's a small checklist. Perhaps you can still do some of these.

Fall in love again. You are certain it can't happen but, oh, it can. Old love (with a sexy older woman) is less taxing than young love but equally stirring.

Experience danger. I took my first hot-air ballooning trip with Malcolm Forbes when I was in my late sixties. My wife, on a dare, decided to swim with the dolphins at the New York Acquarium.

Visit the home of your childhood. I walked through the rooms I knew as a child. The present owners were entranced by my stories—not too long—of what it was like on Long Island in the twenties. They showed me the toy soldiers I had buried there more than sixty years ago.

Call an old flame and have lunch. I took the woman who broke my heart half a century ago to lunch at an old rendezvous on the San Francisco Peninsula and returned her before her husband came home from his office.

Learn to play the piano.

Live in Paris for at least six months.

Start college—or finish it.

Learn Greek.

Visit your parents' graves, with flowers, and think about them for at least an hour while you sit quietly above them.

Do something life-changing for a person or family in need without their knowing you did it.

Buy a painting you love, regardless of how unimportant the artist is.

Change your will in favor of someone you love.

True Truths

I sometimes think the cosmic lessons of life are easily learned, but the lesser lessons are not. Here are a few of my true truths. No doubt you can add some of yours.

Bad news is rarely exaggerated, and first reports of disaster can always be trusted.

A word to the wise is superfluous.

Revenge, as a character in the motion picture *The Sting* rightly says, is for suckers.

Those who don't believe in you won't change their minds when you succeed.

A woman who purses her lips will not approve of drinking, smoking, or the more inventive forms of lovemaking.

A man's attitude toward money is indicative of his meanness or generosity of spirit.

The most unlikely women are the most explosive lovers.

A man's courage can best be judged by what he does when he is without money.

Bad dreams are more likely the result of strong cheeses than suppressed guilt.

114

The most pervasive sadness lies not in growing old but in growing up.

Children have a greater influence on how parents turn out than parents on how children turn out.

A contract that skilled lawyers have labored over for months will turn out not to cover the very points you intended it to cover.

Children can age an adult faster than ten years in prison. Parents can have the same effect on children.

The more attention an executive gives to life-style and perks, the less attention he gives to profits.

Being ruled by what others think of you seldom earns their respect, or yours.

The pursuit of wealth without regard for the limits of personal need or a goal of a more compassionate society is mindless gluttony.

It's Never Too Late for Luck

You can make your luck. "You know what luck is?" says Stanley Kowalski in Tennessee Williams's *A Streetcar Named Desire*. "Luck is believing you're lucky. Take at Salerno. I believed I was lucky. I figured that four out of five would not come through but I would . . . and I did. I put that down as a rule. To hold front position in this rat race you've got to believe you are lucky."

The key to luck is having an optimistic spirit.

The gifted actress Ruth Gordon attributed her success in life and her longevity to following this rule: "Never give up; and never, under any circumstances, no matter what—*never* face the facts."

I've always felt that a certain naïveté—innocence, if you please—prepares you for luck.

I was in my late fifties before I had made any money. My business—films—regarded anyone over forty as a dinosaur and therefore extinct. Twice in my fifties I was jobless, a former top executive reduced to collecting unemployment insurance and sending out résumés. I was terrified of becoming dependent upon a working wife. Successful as she was, she was dependent upon me emotionally. What saved me was my childish refusal, in Ruth Gordon's words, to face facts.

In my personal life I had all the makings of a loser—poorly organized (in fact, sloppy), the product of an unhappy childhood, emotionally insecure, so hungry for affection that I would have married (and did) anyone who showed the slightest tender interest.

How, then, did I meet and marry one of the world's most gifted and, I believe, beautiful women?

I was physically attracted to Helen. She could have had the mental capacity and disposition of a Gila monster, and I would still have been besotted.

It was pure, dumb luck that I had fallen in love with

a bright, devoted, funny, healthy, and talented woman
. . . without knowing she possessed those qualities.
Yet, would it have happened if—after two unsuccess-
ful marriages—I still didn't feel lucky?

Not everyone who feels lucky is lucky. Cancer
strikes. Hearts stop. Planes crash. Loved ones die. It
could happen to me after I write these words. Never
mind. If you cultivate the art of feeling lucky, you have
a better chance to receive its blessing. It's never too
late for luck.

Luck is a lady. If she feels you're interested, she'll
come to you. But she cannot survive naysayers. She
responds only to receptivity and faith. Luck, really, is
no more than an affirmative view of life, a belief in
miracles. And if you do believe, then you can have a
triumphant later life—and a lucky one.

Givens

Some things in life cannot be changed. Instead of
butting your head against the unbeatable or unsolv-
able, walk away.

If you're unlucky with children—and some do grow
up to be beasts—you must divorce them or be wed to
their interminable demands. Don't let the little dar-
lings make you feel guilty. Parenting is not a life
sentence. If it's your life or theirs, choose yours. Their
time on earth is longer.

Some persons are toxic. They poison by their presence or even the timbre of their voices. I have friends

I have known for years but have never really liked. I have no idea why I continued to see them. Perhaps it was like a bad love affair . . . intolerable but unbreakable. Be tougher than I. Unshackle yourself from those you dislike for whatever reason. It's worth the pain of withdrawal.

Avoid put-downers. What a bore to be with a one-upmanship braggart. He or she can do it better, knows it already, was there before you and so on. Don't argue. Slip away.

You must live with the size of your penis, the thinness of your hair, the awkwardness of your gait, the shape of your head. What if you will never move like a gazelle? Walter Duranty, a great foreign correspondent of the Twenties, told a journalist whose leg was smashed, "Think of it this way. Statesmen will say who was the chap with the gimp leg who asked that intelligent question?" Make your signature what you can't hide.

Someday you will lose your grandfather's precious cufflinks. That Ming vase will shatter at your feet. Your wallet containing your driver's license, credit cards, and scads of cash will be lifted. Consider this "breakage." My wife once flushed her antique diamond earring down the toilet and lost the other one in a San Francisco taxi. There's worse "breakage" in life. Death, illness. Forget what can be replaced.

My wife does not agree but I think character or the lack of it can be seen in the face. So can hatefulness. There are beautiful, kind gracious ugly faces and dreadful, cold, cruel beautiful ones. Eventually you look the way you have become, although you started out beautiful as a child.

You will loan money you do not get back. Be glad. An unpaid debt is insurance against lending more. Refuse by calling attention to the unpaid debt.

Those closest—wife, child, parent—are often most difficult to persuade of anything. An acquaintance, passerby or stranger will have more influence.

Arguments are best left unargued. The pleasure of chewing someone out or giving vent to your anger is not worth the anger. Shakespeare had it right. "Those convinced against their will are of the same opinion still."

I'd rather *trust* and be proven misguided than be ruled by suspicion. Those who question every motive and action are unpleasant to be around and usually mistaken.

Run, do not walk, from encounters with irrational or obsessed persons. The mistake is to talk to them as if they were sane.

Don't expect anyone to change. People usually get worse or, at best, stay the way they were. By the way, this is also true of you—and me.

Reprise: Eleven Commandments for Staying Young

Summing up, here are *thou shalts* and *thou shalt nots* according to Brown's Guide. . . . a life plan for staying young gleaned from the chapters you have just read.

1. *Thou shalt not retire.* Work yourself to death—it's the only way to live. Let the young bastards nipping at your heels wait—or find jobs elsewhere. Succession is for sissies.

2. *Thou shalt fool around* (or think about it). Give up sex? Are you mad? Rigor mortis, the final erection, is preferable. Review earlier instructions (chapter two) on how to win your fair share of older women. (Always the best).

3. *Thou shalt marry, though* (but for better, not worse). Wedlock has its compensations—the lock is not one of them. Dump the wrong mate and save yourself. Older women make better wives and are sexually more exciting. Younger women are bad in bed but not bad enough—and also bad for your health. (Ben Franklin's observation). War is hell, but divorce is worse—at first. Later it may be one of the best things you've ever done.

4. *Thou shalt worship thy body.* Get a third, fourth or fifth opinion before contemplating surgery. Your prostate demands sexual activity. Use it or lose it. Never drink when you're tired, tense or angry. The 5 no-no's of Hollywood's health guru to the stars—no booze, no salt, no sugar, no fat, no red meat. You can lengthen your life by starving yourself but eat just enough to fill out those facial wrinkles. Fill up too on those leafy vegetables (cabbage, brussel sprouts) *and* 25 to 35 grams of fiber daily.

5. *Thou shalt not die before thy time.* Death need not be feared. Like Malcolm Forbes, you can *live* until you die—riotously on occasion. Comfort yourself with

the words of William Hazlitt: "There was a time when we were not; this gives us no concern—why, then, should it trouble us that a time will come when we shall cease to be?"

6. *Thou shalt watch thy money.* The best advice ever written about the stock market is to sell when everyone is buying and to buy when everyone is selling. Never invest in a company where you'd be happy as an employee—they probably give away too much. Over-tipping can lengthen your life by reducing stress. Marry a stingy girl—and reform her later. Doctors, especially psychiatrists, are the lousiest investment advisers. Don't try to outlive your money. If you're broke, you'll live forever. If you're rich, you'll die tomorrow. To confound the fates, live it up, but little by little.

7. *Thou shalt not forget.* When you've misplaced a name, run down the alphabet to see if a letter triggers a last name. Retrace your steps when you've lost something of value. Keep double lists of appointments to check against. Never gaze at someone whose name you can't remember—it won't help. You can fake it if trapped into greeting her.

8. *Thou shalt think hopefully.* Nothing prolongs life more than an optimistic attitude. Consider actress Ruth Gordon's advice, "Never give up; and never, under any circumstances, no matter what—*never* face the facts." If you believe in luck, chances are you'll have it.

9. *Thou shalt succeed.* Success is not so much doing what you want as wanting what you do. Success is a man whose children love him and have made him

proud of them. Success is a man who has the love and trust of a woman. Success is a man who does his job superbly and has total control of his life and work. Success is a man who dies at home in his sleep after a good life. Success is what makes you and others feel good. Anything that makes you or others feel bad, regardless of the money you make, is failure.

10. *Thou shalt travel.* It's not only broadening but also life lengthening. An airplane can be better (and cheaper) than a psychiatrist. Travel puts problems in perspective. You can find yourself (or her) when you're lost at sea. (Salt air is an aphrodisiac). The special joys of foreign women . . . live happily with an Italian girl, heartily with a German woman (they *love* older men), extravagantly with a French woman (they can scent a man with money as readily as their dogs can sniff red meat), sensually with a British girl (surprised?).

11. *Thou shalt not want.* Meaning thou shalt not want to be around complainers, crazies, naggers, whiners and other pests. Rid your rolodex of those who blight your life. You actually will live longer without them. Go ahead. Drop them. Be ruthless. They are.